2. Greek Yogurt with Berries and Chia Seeds

Ingredients:
- 1 cup plain Greek yogurt (look for low-fat or non-fat)
- 1/2 cup fresh or frozen mixed berries (such as blueberries, raspberries, strawberries)
- 1 tbsp chia seeds
- 1 tsp honey (optional)
- 1/4 tsp vanilla extract
- 2 tbsp sliced almonds or crushed walnuts

Instructions:

1. In a bowl, gently mix together the Greek yogurt, mixed berries, chia seeds, honey (if using), and vanilla extract until well combined.

2. Top with the sliced almonds or crushed walnuts.

3. Allow to sit for 5-10 minutes so the chia seeds can soften and thicken the yogurt a bit.

4. Enjoy chilled or at room temperature.

Notes:

- Greek yogurt is an excellent source of protein which can aid fertility and help manage PCOS symptoms.

- Berries are low-glycemic, full of antioxidants, and may improve insulin sensitivity.

- Chia seeds provide fiber, protein, and anti-inflammatory omega-3s.

- Honey is a better sweetener than refined sugar for PCOS.

- Almonds and walnuts offer healthy fats and fiber.

- Choose non-fat or low-fat yogurt to reduce calories.

This Greek yogurt parfait makes a nutrient-dense breakfast or snack for those following a PCOS fertility diet. The combination of protein, fiber, antioxidants, and healthy fats may help regulate hormones, periods, and promote ovulation. It's filling while still being low in calories.

3. Spinach and Mushroom Omelet

Ingredients:
- 2 large eggs
- 2 tbsp water or unsweetened almond milk
- 1/4 tsp salt
- 1/4 tsp black pepper
- 1 tsp olive oil or avocado oil
- 1/2 cup fresh baby spinach
- 1/4 cup sliced mushrooms
- 1 tbsp crumbled feta cheese (optional)

Instructions:

1. Crack the eggs into a small bowl and beat them together with the water/milk, salt, and pepper until fully combined.

2. Heat the oil in a small non-stick skillet over medium heat.

3. Add the sliced mushrooms and sauté for 2-3 minutes until tender.

4. Add the spinach and sauté for 1 more minute until the spinach is wilted.

5. Pour in the egg mixture and use a spatula to gently push the cooked egg towards the center as it sets up around the edges.

6. When the bottom is set but the top is still a bit runny, sprinkle the feta cheese (if using) over half of the omelet.

7. Fold the other half over and slide onto a plate. Serve immediately.

Notes:
- Eggs are an excellent source of protein which can aid fertility in PCOS.
- Spinach provides antioxidants, folate, and helps reduce inflammation.
- Mushrooms are rich in vitamin D which supports reproductive health.
- Feta adds flavor but can be omitted or substituted for alternative dairy.
- Cook with olive oil or avocado oil instead of butter.
- For extra fiber, serve with a slice of whole grain toast.

This protein-packed omelet supplies key nutrients like folate, antioxidants, and vitamin D that are beneficial for PCOS fertility. It makes a satisfying and nutritious start to the day for women trying to conceive with PCOS.

Introduction

Living with Polycystic Ovary Syndrome (PCOS) can be challenging, especially when it comes to managing symptoms and enhancing fertility. For many women, the journey through PCOS involves navigating a myriad of symptoms such as irregular menstrual cycles, hormonal imbalances, weight fluctuations, and insulin resistance. These challenges not only affect physical health but also take a toll on emotional and mental well-being. Understanding the pivotal role that diet and nutrition play in managing PCOS can empower women to take control of their health and improve their chances of conceiving.

Welcome to the ***"PCOS Fertility Diet Cookbook for Women: Nutrient-Rich Meals for Balancing Hormones and Enhancing Fertility".*** This book is designed to be a comprehensive guide that blends the latest scientific research with practical, delicious, and easy-to-prepare recipes aimed at addressing the unique nutritional needs of women with PCOS.

In this cookbook, you will find a wealth of information about how specific nutrients and foods can help balance hormones, improve insulin sensitivity, and support overall reproductive health. Whether you are newly diagnosed or have been managing PCOS for years, the recipes and meal plans in this book are crafted to support you on your journey toward better health and fertility.

Each recipe is carefully developed to provide essential nutrients that are often lacking in the typical diet of someone with PCOS. You will discover meals that are rich in fiber, lean proteins, healthy fats, and low-glycemic carbohydrates, all of which are crucial for maintaining stable blood sugar levels and hormonal balance. Additionally, the recipes focus on whole, unprocessed foods to ensure you are getting the most nutritional benefit from every bite.

We also understand that time and convenience are important, especially for women balancing busy lives. Therefore, the recipes in this cookbook are designed to be simple and quick, without sacrificing flavor or nutrition. From hearty breakfasts and satisfying lunches to nourishing dinners and tasty snacks, you will find a variety of meals that fit seamlessly into your lifestyle.

This cookbook is more than just a collection of recipes; it is a resource for education and empowerment. Throughout the book, you will find tips on meal planning, grocery shopping, and mindful eating, as well as insights into how different foods and nutrients impact your body. By making informed dietary choices, you can take proactive steps toward managing PCOS and enhancing your fertility.

Embark on this culinary journey with us and discover how the right foods can transform your health. Let the "PCOS Fertility Diet Cookbook for Women" be your guide to balanced hormones, improved fertility, and a healthier, happier you.

1. Avocado Toast with Whole Grain Bread

Ingredients:
- 1/2 cup old-fashioned rolled oats
- 1 cup unsweetened almond milk or low-fat milk
- 1/2 cup fresh or frozen blueberries
- 1 tbsp honey
- 1 tsp ground cinnamon
- 1/4 tsp vanilla extract
- 1 tbsp chopped walnuts or almonds (optional)

Instructions:

1. In a small saucepan, combine the oats and milk. Bring to a gentle boil over medium heat.

2. Reduce heat to low and simmer for 5-7 minutes, stirring frequently, until oats are tender and creamy.

3. Remove from heat and stir in the blueberries, honey, cinnamon, and vanilla extract until well combined.

4. Transfer oatmeal to a bowl and top with chopped nuts (if using). Serve warm.

Notes:

- Oats are high in fiber which can help improve insulin resistance in PCOS. The soluble fiber also promotes healthy gut bacteria.

- Blueberries are low-glycemic and packed with antioxidants that may improve insulin sensitivity.

- Honey is a better sweetener option than refined sugar for PCOS.

- Cinnamon helps regulate blood sugar levels.

- Unsweetened almond milk is low in calories and won't spike insulin levels.

- Walnuts or almonds provide healthy fats and protein to keep you full longer.

This comforting and nutritious oatmeal breakfast fits well into a PCOS fertility diet. It's high in fiber, antioxidants and features low-glycemic ingredients to help manage insulin resistance and promote ovulation.

4. Quinoa Porridge with Almond Milk and Fresh Fruit

Ingredients:
- 1 cup cooked quinoa
- 1 1/2 cups unsweetened almond milk
- 1 tsp ground cinnamon
- 1/4 tsp vanilla extract
- 2 tbsp slivered almonds or chopped walnuts
- 1 cup fresh fruit (berries, diced mango, sliced banana etc.)
- 1-2 tsp honey or maple syrup (optional)

Instructions:

1. In a small saucepan, combine the cooked quinoa and almond milk. Bring to a gentle simmer over medium heat, stirring occasionally.

2. Once simmering, reduce heat to low and continue cooking for 5-7 minutes, stirring frequently, until thickened to a porridge-like consistency.

3. Remove from heat and stir in the cinnamon and vanilla extract until well combined.

4. Divide the warm quinoa porridge between two bowls. Top each with fresh fruit, slivered almonds/walnuts, and a drizzle of honey/maple syrup if desired.

Notes:
- Quinoa is a protein-rich grain that is high in fiber to help manage PCOS symptoms.

- Almond milk is dairy-free, low in calories, and won't spike insulin levels.

- Cinnamon helps regulate blood sugar levels.

- Fresh fruit provides antioxidants, but stick to low-glycemic options like berries.

- Nuts offer healthy fats and plant-based protein.

- Honey is a better sweetener option than refined sugar for PCOS.

This quinoa porridge bowl makes a delicious and nourishing PCOS-friendly breakfast. It's packed with protein, fiber, antioxidants and healthy fats to promote insulin sensitivity and ovulation. The warm, comforting porridge with fresh fruit is also very satisfying.

5. Overnight Oats with Flaxseeds and Blueberries

Ingredients:
- 1/2 cup old-fashioned rolled oats
- 1/2 cup unsweetened almond milk or low-fat milk
- 1/4 cup plain Greek yogurt
- 1 tbsp ground flaxseeds
- 1 tsp honey or maple syrup (optional)
- 1/2 tsp vanilla extract
- 1/2 cup fresh or frozen blueberries
- 1 tbsp chopped walnuts or almonds

Instructions:

1. In a mason jar or bowl, combine the rolled oats, almond milk, Greek yogurt, flaxseeds, honey/maple syrup (if using), and vanilla. Stir well until fully mixed.

2. Gently fold in half of the blueberries.

3. Cover and refrigerate overnight (or for at least 6 hours).

4. In the morning, remove from fridge and give it a stir. Top with the remaining blueberries and chopped nuts. Optionally, heat up for 30-60 seconds in the microwave if you prefer it warm.

Notes:
- Oats are high in soluble fiber to help regulate periods and improve insulin resistance in PCOS.

- Greek yogurt provides protein which aids fertility.

- Flaxseeds are high in lignans that can help balance hormones.

- Blueberries are antioxidant-rich and low-glycemic.

- Nuts offer healthy fats and plant protein.

- Use unsweetened non-dairy milk or low-fat dairy milk. Honey is a better sweetener than refined sugar for PCOS.

These make-ahead overnight oats are perfect for a quick, nutritious PCOS fertility diet breakfast. The fiber, protein, antioxidants, and omega-3s may improve insulin sensitivity, reduce inflammation, and promote ovulation. Customize with your favorite nut butter or fruit too.

6. Smoothie with Spinach, Banana, and Almond Butter

Ingredients:
- 1 cup unsweetened almond milk or low-fat milk
- 1 banana
- 1 cup fresh baby spinach
- 2 tbsp almond butter
- 1 tsp ground flaxseeds
- 1/2 tsp ground cinnamon
- 1/2 tsp vanilla extract
- 2-3 ice cubes

Instructions:

1. Add the almond milk, banana, spinach, almond butter, flaxseeds, cinnamon, and vanilla to a blender.

2. Blend on high speed until completely smooth and no chunks remain, about 1 minute.

3. Add the ice cubes and blend again briefly until they are crushed and the smoothie is thick and frosty.

4. Pour into a glass and enjoy immediately.

Notes:
- Spinach is nutrient-dense and provides folate, iron and antioxidants for PCOS.

- Banana adds sweetness, fiber, and healthy carbs.

- Almond butter offers protein, healthy fats, and vitamin E.

- Flaxseeds are rich in lignans that help balance hormones.

- Cinnamon helps regulate blood sugar levels.

- Use unsweetened non-dairy milk or low-fat dairy milk.

This creamy green smoothie packs in plenty of PCOS-friendly nutrients like protein, fiber, antioxidants and plant-based omega-3s. It makes a nutritious on-the-go breakfast or snack for women trying to conceive with PCOS. The healthy fats, antioxidants and fiber may improve insulin resistance, ovulation and fertility.

7. Scrambled Tofu with Vegetables

Ingredients:
- 1 (14 oz) block firm or extra-firm tofu, drained and crumbled
- 2 tsp olive oil or avocado oil
- 1 cup sliced mushrooms
- 1 cup baby spinach
- 1/2 bell pepper, diced
- 1/4 cup diced onion
- 1 clove garlic, minced
- 1/4 tsp turmeric
- 1/4 tsp cumin
- Salt and pepper to taste
- 1 tbsp nutritional yeast (optional)
- Chopped green onions or herbs for garnish

Instructions:
1. In a non-stick skillet, heat the oil over medium heat. Add the mushrooms, bell pepper, onion and garlic. Sauté for 3-4 minutes until vegetables are tender.

2. Crumble the tofu into the skillet and mix with the vegetables.

3. Sprinkle in the turmeric, cumin, salt and pepper. Stir to combine.

4. Add in the baby spinach and continue cooking for 2-3 more minutes until spinach is wilted and tofu is heated through.

5. Remove from heat and stir in nutritional yeast if using.

6. Garnish with chopped green onions or fresh herbs if desired.

Notes:
- Tofu is an excellent source of protein and antioxidants beneficial for PCOS fertility.
- Mushrooms provide vitamin D which supports reproductive health.
- Leafy greens like spinach offer folate, iron and antioxidants.
- Turmeric may help reduce inflammation associated with PCOS.
- Olive oil or avocado oil provide healthy fats.
- Nutritional yeast adds a savory, cheesy flavor and B-vitamins.

This high-protein, veggie-packed scrambled tofu makes a delicious and nutritious savory breakfast or lunch for women with PCOS trying to conceive. It's full of fertility-boosting nutrients to potentially improve insulin resistance and ovulation.

8. Chia Seed Pudding with Almond Milk and Raspberries

Ingredients:
- 1/4 cup chia seeds
- 1 cup unsweetened almond milk
- 1/2 tsp vanilla extract
- 1-2 tsp honey or maple syrup (optional)
- 1 cup fresh or frozen raspberries
- 2 tbsp sliced almonds

Instructions:

1. In a bowl or mason jar, combine the chia seeds, almond milk, vanilla extract and honey/maple syrup if using. Whisk well to prevent clumping.

2. Cover and refrigerate for at least 2 hours or overnight to allow the chia seeds to swell and thicken into a pudding-like consistency.

3. Once thickened, give it a stir and divide the chia pudding between two bowls or jars.

4. Top each serving with 1/2 cup fresh or frozen raspberries and 1 tbsp sliced almonds.

Notes:

- Chia seeds are high in fiber, protein, antioxidants and omega-3s beneficial for PCOS.

- Almond milk is dairy-free, low in calories and won't spike insulin.

- Raspberries are high in fiber, antioxidants and have a low glycemic index.

- Honey or maple syrup add sweetness without refined sugar.

- Almonds provide healthy fats, protein and crunch.

This make-ahead chia pudding makes a perfect PCOS-friendly breakfast or snack. The chia seeds help regulate blood sugar while the berries provide antioxidants. The healthy fats and protein from the nuts and seeds also aid fertility and ovulation for PCOS. It's nutritious and satisfying.

9. Whole Grain Pancakes with Mixed Berries

Ingredients:
- 1 cup whole wheat flour or oat flour
- 1 tsp baking powder
- 1/2 tsp baking soda
- 1/4 tsp salt
- 1 cup unsweetened almond milk
- 1 egg
- 1 tbsp honey or maple syrup
- 1 tsp vanilla extract
- 1 cup mixed fresh or frozen berries (blueberries, raspberries, blackberries)
- Butter or oil for cooking

Instructions:
1. In a large bowl, whisk together the whole wheat/oat flour, baking powder, baking soda and salt.

2. In a separate bowl, whisk together the almond milk, egg, honey/maple syrup and vanilla.

3. Pour the wet ingredients into the dry ingredients and mix just until combined (don't overmix).

4. Heat a non-stick griddle or skillet over medium heat and grease lightly with butter or oil.

5. For each pancake, pour about 1/4 cup of batter onto the hot griddle. Sprinkle some berries over the top of each pancake.

6. Cook for 2-3 minutes per side until golden brown, flipping carefully.

7. Serve the pancakes warm with extra berries, a drizzle of maple syrup or honey if desired.

Notes:
- Whole grains provide fiber to help regulate blood sugar levels.
- Berries are low-glycemic, high in antioxidants and may improve insulin sensitivity.
- Eggs offer protein to aid fertility in PCOS.
- Almond milk is dairy-free and low in calories.
- Honey or maple syrup are better sweetener choices than refined sugar.

These fluffy whole grain pancakes make a delicious PCOS fertility diet breakfast. The fiber from the whole grains along with antioxidant-rich berries may improve insulin resistance and promote ovulation. Top with nut butter for extra protein too!

10. Cottage Cheese with Pineapple and Walnuts

Ingredients:
- 1 cup low-fat cottage cheese
- 1/2 cup fresh pineapple chunks
- 2 tbsp chopped walnuts
- 1 tsp ground cinnamon
- 1 tsp honey (optional)

Instructions:

1. In a bowl, combine the cottage cheese, fresh pineapple chunks, and chopped walnuts.

2. Sprinkle the cinnamon over the top and gently fold everything together until well mixed.

3. Drizzle with 1 tsp of honey if desired for a touch of sweetness.

4. Enjoy chilled or at room temperature.

Notes:

- Cottage cheese is an excellent source of protein which aids fertility in PCOS.

- Pineapple is rich in antioxidants like vitamin C and bromelain which may help reduce inflammation.

- Walnuts provide healthy omega-3 fatty acids and fiber.

- Cinnamon helps regulate blood sugar levels.

- Honey is a better sweetener option than refined sugar for PCOS.

This cottage cheese bowl makes a nutritious and satisfying snack or light meal for women with PCOS. The protein, antioxidants, healthy fats and fiber may help improve insulin resistance, ovulation and fertility. The touch of sweetness from the pineapple and cinnamon adds great flavor too.

11. Apple Slices with Almond Butter

Ingredients:
- 1 medium apple, sliced
- 2 tbsp natural almond butter
- 1 tsp honey (optional)
- Pinch of cinnamon
- 1 tbsp chopped walnuts or almonds

Instructions:
1. Wash the apple and slice it into wedges or thin slices, removing the core.

2. Spread or dip the apple slices into the almond butter.

3. If desired, drizzle a teaspoon of honey over the almond butter coated apple slices.

4. Sprinkle with a pinch of cinnamon.

5. Top with chopped walnuts or almonds.

Notes:

- Apples are high in fiber to help regulate blood sugar levels for PCOS.

- Almond butter provides healthy fats, protein, and vitamin E beneficial for fertility.

- Honey is a better sweetener choice than refined sugar for PCOS.

- Cinnamon helps improve insulin sensitivity.

- Walnuts and almonds add crunch and offer additional healthy fats and nutrients.

This simple snack combines fiber, protein, healthy fats, and antioxidants - all nutrients that may help improve PCOS symptoms and boost fertility. The almond butter provides lasting satiety, while the apple and nuts offer fiber to prevent blood sugar spikes. It's a delicious and nutritious PCOS-friendly snack or dessert option.

12. Carrot and Cucumber Sticks with Hummus

Ingredients:
- 4 medium carrots, peeled and cut into sticks
- 1 large cucumber, cut into sticks
- 1 (15oz) can chickpeas, drained and rinsed
- 2 tbsp tahini
- 2 tbsp lemon juice
- 1 garlic clove, minced
- 2 tbsp olive oil
- 1/4 cup water
- 1/2 tsp cumin
- Salt and pepper to taste
- Chopped parsley for garnish

Instructions:

1. Make the hummus by adding the chickpeas, tahini, lemon juice, garlic, olive oil, water and cumin to a food processor or blender. Season with salt and pepper.

2. Process/blend until smooth and creamy, scraping down sides as needed. Add more water a tablespoon at a time if too thick.

3. Transfer hummus to a bowl. Drizzle with a bit of olive oil and sprinkle parsley over the top.

4. Arrange the carrot and cucumber sticks around the hummus for dipping.

Notes:
- Carrots and cucumbers provide antioxidants, fiber, and a crunchy veggie dipping option.

- Chickpeas in the hummus offer protein, fiber and nutrients to support PCOS.

- Tahini (sesame seed butter) provides healthy fats and minerals like calcium.

- Olive oil adds anti-inflammatory monounsaturated fats.

- Cumin and other spices/herbs add flavor without salt or sugar.

This veggie platter with protein-packed hummus makes a nutritious PCOS-friendly snack or appetizer. The fiber from the veggies and chickpeas may help regulate blood sugar. The healthy fats promote hormone balance and fertility. The simple ingredients avoid processed foods/sugars that could exacerbate PCOS symptoms.

13. Mixed Nuts and Seeds

Ingredients:
- 1/2 cup raw almonds
- 1/2 cup raw walnuts
- 1/4 cup raw pumpkin seeds
- 1/4 cup raw sunflower seeds
- 2 tbsp chia seeds
- 1 tbsp ground flaxseeds
- 1 tsp olive oil or avocado oil
- 1/2 tsp ground cinnamon
- 1/4 tsp salt (optional)

Instructions:

1. Preheat oven to 325°F (165°C). Line a baking sheet with parchment paper.

2. In a bowl, combine the almonds, walnuts, pumpkin seeds, sunflower seeds, chia seeds and ground flaxseeds.

3. Drizzle with the oil and sprinkle with cinnamon and salt (if using). Toss to coat evenly.

4. Spread the nut and seed mixture in a single layer on the prepared baking sheet.

5. Bake for 12-15 minutes, stirring halfway, until lightly toasted and fragrant.

6. Allow to cool completely before transferring to an airtight container.

Notes:

- Nuts and seeds provide protein, healthy fats, fiber and minerals like zinc to support PCOS.

- Almonds and walnuts offer anti-inflammatory omega-3s.

- Pumpkin and sunflower seeds are rich in zinc which aids ovulation.

- Chia and flaxseeds supply fiber and lignans to help balance hormones.

- Cinnamon helps regulate blood sugar levels.

- Roasting with oil and spices adds flavor and crunch.

- Portion into 1/4 cup servings for a PCOS-friendly snack or salad topper.

This nutritious mixed nut and seed blend provides an array of fertility-boosting nutrients for women with PCOS. The protein, healthy fats, fiber and antioxidants may improve insulin resistance, reduce inflammation and promote ovulation. It makes a satisfying and portable snack.

14. Edamame with Sea Salt

Ingredients:
- 1 lb (454g) frozen edamame in pods
- 1 tsp sea salt or kosher salt
- 2 tsp olive oil or avocado oil (optional)

Instructions:
1. Bring a pot of water to a boil over high heat. Add the frozen edamame.

2. Once the water returns to a boil, reduce heat to medium and simmer for 5 minutes.

3. Drain the edamame in a colander and rinse with cool water to stop the cooking process.

4. Transfer the cooked edamame to a bowl. Drizzle with olive oil or avocado oil if desired.

5. Sprinkle with sea salt or kosher salt and toss to coat evenly.

6. Serve warm or at room temperature.

Notes:
- Edamame is the young soybeans packed with protein, fiber, antioxidants and folate.

- Protein aids fertility and helps manage PCOS symptoms like insulin resistance.

- Folate is important for reproductive health and prevents birth defects.

- Sea salt provides sodium and minerals without adding refined salt.

- Olive or avocado oil adds healthy monounsaturated fats.

- For extra flavor, sprinkle with chili powder, garlic powder or lemon juice.

Edamame makes an excellent PCOS-friendly snack or appetizer. The plant-based protein and fiber help regulate blood sugar levels, while the folate and antioxidants support ovulation and fertility. It's a simple, nutritious option that may improve hormonal imbalances related to PCOS.

15. Greek Yogurt with Honey and Almonds

Ingredients:
- 1 cup plain Greek yogurt (non-fat or low-fat)
- 2 tsp honey
- 2 tbsp sliced or slivered almonds
- 1/2 tsp vanilla extract (optional)
- Pinch of cinnamon (optional)

Instructions:
1. In a bowl, scoop out 1 cup of plain Greek yogurt.

2. Drizzle the honey over the yogurt.

3. Sprinkle the sliced or slivered almonds over the top.

4. If desired, add 1/2 tsp vanilla extract and a pinch of cinnamon. Gently mix everything together.

5. Enjoy chilled or at room temperature.

Notes:
- Greek yogurt provides protein which aids fertility and manages PCOS symptoms.

- Choose non-fat or low-fat varieties to reduce calories.

- Honey is a better sweetener option than refined sugar for PCOS.

- Almonds offer healthy fats, fiber, and plant-based protein.

- Cinnamon may help regulate blood sugar levels.

- For extra antioxidants, top with fresh berries or pomegranate seeds.

This protein-packed yogurt snack or dessert contains PCOS-friendly ingredients like Greek yogurt, nuts, and honey. The protein may improve insulin resistance while the healthy fats promote hormone balance. The touch of honey adds sweetness without spiking blood sugar levels. It's a simple yet nutritious option for women with PCOS trying to conceive.

16. Baked Kale Chips

Ingredients:
- 1 large bundle kale (about 10 cups chopped)
- 1 tbsp olive oil or avocado oil
- 1/2 tsp garlic powder
- 1/4 tsp salt
- 1/4 tsp black pepper

Instructions:
1. Preheat oven to 300°F (150°C). Line 2 large baking sheets with parchment paper.

2. Remove kale leaves from the thick stems and roughly tear into bite-sized pieces. Wash and thoroughly dry the kale (use a salad spinner if possible).

3. Transfer the kale leaves to a large bowl. Drizzle with oil and use your hands to massage the oil into the leaves until fully coated.

4. Sprinkle the garlic powder, salt, and black pepper over the kale. Toss to evenly distribute the seasonings.

5. Arrange the kale in a single layer on the prepared baking sheets, being careful not to overcrowd.

6. Bake for 18-22 minutes, rotating the pans halfway, until crispy but not browned.

7. Remove from oven and allow to cool completely on the baking sheets before serving.

Notes:
- Kale is rich in antioxidants, fiber, iron, and folate to support PCOS fertility.
- Olive or avocado oil provide healthy fats without refined oils.
- Garlic powder and other spices add flavor without salt or sugar.
- For variety, use different seasoning like chili powder, curry powder, nutritional yeast.
- Bake until crispy but avoid browning to prevent bitterness.
- Let cool fully before eating for maximum crunch.

These crispy baked kale chips make a nutritious PCOS-friendly snack or side dish. The antioxidants and fiber may help regulate blood sugar and reduce inflammation associated with PCOS. The simple kale chips are low-calorie yet filling and packed with fertility-boosting nutrients.

17. Fresh Fruit Salad

Ingredients:
- 1 cup fresh strawberries, sliced
- 1 cup fresh blueberries
- 1 cup fresh raspberries
- 1 cup fresh pineapple chunks
- 1 kiwi fruit, peeled and sliced
- 1 tbsp honey
- 2 tbsp fresh lime juice
- 1 tsp lime zest
- Mint leaves for garnish (optional)

Instructions:

1. In a large bowl, gently combine the strawberries, blueberries, raspberries, pineapple chunks, and kiwi slices.

2. In a small bowl, whisk together the honey, lime juice, and lime zest until well combined.

3. Drizzle the honey-lime dressing over the fruit salad and gently toss to coat the fruits evenly.

4. Garnish with mint leaves (if desired).

5. Refrigerate for at least 30 minutes before serving to allow the flavors to blend.

This fresh fruit salad is not only delicious but also packed with essential nutrients that can benefit women with PCOS. It's rich in antioxidants, fiber, and various vitamins and minerals that support overall health and fertility. Additionally, the honey provides a natural sweetness while being a better alternative to refined sugars.

Enjoy this refreshing and nutritious fruit salad as a snack, dessert, or a side dish as part of a balanced PCOS fertility diet.

18. Rice Cakes with Avocado and Tomato

Ingredients:
- 4 brown rice cakes
- 1 ripe avocado, mashed
- 1 tomato, diced
- 1 tablespoon fresh lemon juice
- 1 tablespoon extra-virgin olive oil
- 1/4 teaspoon sea salt
- 1/4 teaspoon black pepper
- 1/4 cup fresh basil leaves, chopped (optional)

Instructions:
1. In a small bowl, mash the avocado with a fork until it reaches a smooth, creamy consistency.

2. Add the diced tomato, lemon juice, olive oil, sea salt, and black pepper to the mashed avocado. Mix well until combined.

3. Toast the brown rice cakes according to package instructions or until slightly crispy.

4. Spread the avocado mixture evenly over the toasted rice cakes.

5. Sprinkle the chopped fresh basil leaves over the top (if using).

Benefits for PCOS Fertility Diet:
1. Brown rice cakes: Provide complex carbohydrates, which are essential for maintaining balanced blood sugar levels, a crucial factor in managing PCOS.

2. Avocado: Rich in healthy monounsaturated fats, which can help improve insulin sensitivity and promote regular ovulation.

3. Tomato: A good source of antioxidants, such as lycopene, which may help reduce inflammation associated with PCOS.

4. Lemon juice: Provides vitamin C, which supports overall fertility and may improve insulin resistance in women with PCOS.

5. Olive oil: A source of healthy fats and antioxidants, which can benefit overall reproductive health.

6. Fresh basil: Offers additional antioxidants and may help improve insulin sensitivity.

This snack or light meal is not only delicious but also provides a good balance of nutrients that can support fertility in women with PCOS. It's a convenient and satisfying option that can be enjoyed anytime.

19. Celery Sticks with Peanut Butter

Ingredients:

- 6-8 celery sticks, washed and trimmed
- 1/4 cup natural peanut butter (look for a brand with no added sugars or oils)
- 1 tablespoon ground flaxseeds (optional)

Instructions:

1. Wash and trim the celery sticks, cutting them into desired lengths.

2. Spread a generous amount of natural peanut butter onto each celery stick.

3. If desired, sprinkle ground flaxseeds over the peanut butter for an added nutritional boost.

Benefits for PCOS Fertility Diet:

1. Celery: Low in calories and high in fiber, celery can help promote a feeling of fullness and support weight management, which is important for managing PCOS.

2. Peanut butter: A good source of protein and healthy fats, both of which are essential for hormone regulation and fertility. The protein in peanut butter can also help stabilize blood sugar levels.

3. Ground flaxseeds (optional): Flaxseeds are rich in omega-3 fatty acids, fiber, and lignans, which may help improve insulin sensitivity and reduce inflammation associated with PCOS.

This snack is not only convenient and easy to prepare but also provides essential nutrients that can benefit women with PCOS. The combination of celery, peanut butter, and flaxseeds (if using) can help regulate blood sugar levels, improve insulin sensitivity, and reduce inflammation, all of which are important factors in managing PCOS and supporting fertility.

Additionally, the fiber and protein in this snack can help promote a feeling of fullness, which can aid in weight management, another important aspect of managing PCOS.

Enjoy this satisfying and nutritious snack as part of a balanced PCOS fertility diet.

20. Hard-Boiled Eggs

Nutritional Benefits:

1. Protein: Eggs are an excellent source of high-quality protein, which is crucial for hormone regulation and fertility. Adequate protein intake can help manage insulin resistance, a common issue in women with PCOS.

2. Choline: Eggs are one of the richest dietary sources of choline, an essential nutrient that plays a vital role in fetal brain development and may improve fertility outcomes.

3. Vitamin D: Eggs contain small amounts of vitamin D, which is important for reproductive health and may help regulate menstrual cycles in women with PCOS.

4. Selenium: Eggs are a good source of selenium, an antioxidant mineral that may help reduce inflammation and improve insulin sensitivity, both of which are important for managing PCOS.

5. Zinc: Eggs provide zinc, a mineral that plays a role in hormone regulation and fertility. Zinc deficiency has been associated with PCOS and may contribute to irregular menstrual cycles.

6. Low in carbohydrates: Hard-boiled eggs are naturally low in carbohydrates, making them a suitable choice for women with PCOS who may need to follow a low-carb or low-glycemic diet to manage insulin resistance.

Preparation and Serving Suggestions:
Hard-boiled eggs are incredibly versatile and can be enjoyed in various ways, such as:

- On their own as a snack
- Added to salads for extra protein
- Served with avocado or hummus for a more substantial meal
- Incorporated into egg salad or egg sandwiches

To prepare hard-boiled eggs, simply place eggs in a saucepan, cover with water, and bring to a boil. Remove from heat, cover, and let stand for 12-15 minutes. Drain and cool the eggs before peeling and enjoying.

By incorporating hard-boiled eggs into your PCOS fertility diet, you can benefit from their nutritional value and support overall reproductive health. Remember to enjoy them as part of a balanced diet and consult with a healthcare professional for personalized dietary recommendations.

21. Grilled Chicken Salad with Mixed Greens and Olive Oil Dressing

Ingredients:
For the dressing:
- 3 tablespoons extra-virgin olive oil
- 2 tablespoons red wine
vinegar or lemon juice
- 1 teaspoon Dijon mustard
- 1 clove garlic, minced
- Salt and pepper to taste

For the salad:
- 2 boneless, skinless chicken breasts
- 1 teaspoon olive oil
- Salt and pepper to taste
- 4 cups mixed greens (e.g., spinach, arugula, romaine lettuce)
- 1 cup cherry tomatoes, halved
- 1/2 cucumber, sliced
- 1/4 red onion, thinly sliced

Instructions:
1. Preheat your grill or grill pan to medium-high heat.

2. Brush the chicken breasts with 1 teaspoon of olive oil and season with salt and pepper.

3. Grill the chicken breasts for about 6-8 minutes per side, or until cooked through and no longer pink in the center. Let them rest for 5 minutes before slicing.

4. While the chicken is grilling, prepare the dressing by whisking together the olive oil, red wine vinegar (or lemon juice), Dijon mustard, minced garlic, salt, and pepper in a small bowl.

5. In a large salad bowl, combine the mixed greens, cherry tomatoes, cucumber slices, and red onion slices.

6. Slice the grilled chicken breasts and add them to the salad bowl. Drizzle the olive oil dressing over the salad and gently toss to coat all the ingredients evenly.

Benefits for PCOS Fertility Diet:
1. Lean protein: Grilled chicken is an excellent source of lean protein, which is essential for maintaining balanced blood sugar levels and promoting regular ovulation in women with PCOS.

2. Fiber-rich greens: The mixed greens in this salad provide a good source of fiber, which can help improve insulin sensitivity and promote healthy digestion.

3. Healthy fats: The olive oil in the dressing provides heart-healthy monounsaturated fats, which may help improve insulin sensitivity and reduce inflammation associated with PCOS.

4. Antioxidants: The vegetables in the salad, such as tomatoes and onions, are rich in antioxidants that can help combat oxidative stress and inflammation, both of which are linked to PCOS

22. Quinoa and Black Bean Salad

Ingredients:
- 1 cup uncooked quinoa
- 1 (15 oz) can black beans, rinsed and drained
- 1 red bell pepper, diced
- 1 cup cherry tomatoes, halved
- 1/2 red onion, diced
- 1/4 cup fresh cilantro, chopped
- 2 tablespoons extra-virgin olive oil
- 2 tablespoons lime juice
- 1 teaspoon cumin
- 1/2 teaspoon chili powder
- Salt and pepper to taste

Instructions:

1. Cook the quinoa according to package instructions. Once cooked, fluff it with a fork and let it cool completely.

2. In a large bowl, combine the cooked and cooled quinoa, rinsed black beans, diced red bell pepper, halved cherry tomatoes, diced red onion, and chopped cilantro.

3. In a small bowl, whisk together the olive oil, lime juice, cumin, chili powder, salt, and pepper to make the dressing.

4. Pour the dressing over the quinoa and black bean mixture and toss gently to combine. Taste and adjust seasoning if needed.

5. Refrigerate the salad for at least 30 minutes to allow the flavors to meld together before serving.

Benefits for PCOS Fertility Diet:

1. Quinoa: A nutrient-dense whole grain that provides complex carbohydrates, fiber, and protein, all of which can help regulate blood sugar levels and promote insulin sensitivity in women with PCOS.

2. Black beans: An excellent source of plant-based protein, fiber, and various vitamins and minerals, such as iron and folate, which are important for fertility.

3. Fresh vegetables: The bell pepper, tomatoes, and onion provide antioxidants, vitamins, and fiber, which can help reduce inflammation and support overall health.

4. Olive oil: A source of healthy monounsaturated fats, which may help improve insulin sensitivity and reduce the risk of metabolic complications associated with PCOS.

5. Lime juice and spices: The lime juice, cumin, and chili powder add a zesty flavor while providing additional antioxidants and anti-inflammatory properties.

23. Lentil Soup with Vegetables

Ingredients:
- 1 cup dry lentils (green or brown), rinsed
- 1 tablespoon olive oil
- 1 onion, diced
- 2 carrots, diced
- 2 celery stalks, diced
- 3 cloves garlic, minced
- 1 teaspoon ground cumin
- 1/2 teaspoon dried thyme
- 6 cups vegetable or chicken broth
- 1 (14.5 oz) can diced tomatoes
- 2 cups chopped kale or spinach
- Salt and pepper to taste
- Lemon wedges for serving (optional)

Instructions:

1. In a large pot or Dutch oven, heat the olive oil over medium heat.

2. Add the diced onion, carrots, and celery. Sauté for about 5 minutes until the vegetables start to soften. Add the minced garlic, cumin, and dried thyme. Cook for another minute, stirring constantly.

3. Add the rinsed lentils, vegetable or chicken broth, and diced tomatoes (with their juices) to the pot.

4. Bring the soup to a boil, then reduce the heat to low and let it simmer for 20-25 minutes, or until the lentils are tender. Stir in the chopped kale or spinach and let it wilt for a few minutes.

5. Season the soup with salt and pepper to taste. Serve hot, optionally with a squeeze of fresh lemon juice.

Benefits for PCOS Fertility Diet:

1. Lentils: A great source of plant-based protein, fiber, and complex carbohydrates, which can help regulate blood sugar levels and improve insulin sensitivity in women with PCOS.

2. Vegetables: The combination of carrots, celery, onions, garlic, and leafy greens (kale or spinach) provides a wealth of vitamins, minerals, and antioxidants that can support overall health and fertility.

3. Olive oil: A source of healthy monounsaturated fats, which may help improve insulin sensitivity and reduce inflammation associated with PCOS.

This lentil soup with vegetables is not only delicious and comforting but also packed with essential nutrients that can support fertility and overall health in women with PCOS. It's a filling and satisfying meal that can be enjoyed for lunch or dinner, providing a balanced combination of protein, complex carbohydrates, fiber, and various vitamins and minerals. Enjoy it as part of a well-rounded PCOS fertility diet.

24. Turkey and Avocado Wrap in Whole Wheat Tortilla

Ingredients:
- 1 whole wheat tortilla
- 3-4 slices of roasted turkey breast (nitrate-free)
- 1/4 avocado, sliced
- 1/4 cup shredded lettuce
- 1/4 cup sliced cucumber
- 1/4 cup shredded carrots
- 2 tablespoons hummus (optional)
- Salt and pepper to taste

Instructions:
1. Lay the whole wheat tortilla flat on a clean surface.

2. Spread a layer of hummus (if using) evenly over the tortilla.

3. Place the roasted turkey slices evenly over the hummus.

4. Arrange the avocado slices, shredded lettuce, sliced cucumber, and shredded carrots over the turkey.

5. Season with salt and pepper to taste.

6. Carefully roll up the tortilla, tucking in the sides as you go, to form a wrap.

7. Slice the wrap in half diagonally. Serve immediately or wrap tightly in foil or parchment paper for later.

Nutritional Benefits:
- ***Whole Wheat Tortilla:*** Provides complex carbohydrates and fiber, which can help stabilize blood sugar levels.

- ***Turkey:*** A lean source of protein that can help support muscle health.

- ***Avocado:*** Rich in healthy fats and fiber, which can help regulate hormones and promote fertility.

- ***Vegetables:*** Provide essential vitamins, minerals, and antioxidants for overall health.

- ***Hummus (optional):*** Adds extra flavor and creaminess, and also provides plant-based protein and fiber.

25. Spinach and Feta Stuffed Bell Peppers

Ingredients:
- 4 large bell peppers (any color)
- 2 cups fresh spinach, chopped
- 1 cup cooked quinoa
- 1/2 cup crumbled feta cheese
- 1/4 cup chopped red onion
- 2 cloves garlic, minced
- 1 tablespoon olive oil
- 1 teaspoon dried oregano
- Salt and pepper to taste
- 1/4 cup chopped fresh parsley (optional, for garnish)

Instructions:

1. Preheat your oven to 375°F (190°C).

2. Cut the tops off the bell peppers and remove the seeds and membranes. If needed, trim the bottom slightly so they stand upright.

3. In a large skillet, heat the olive oil over medium heat. Add the chopped red onion and cook until it becomes translucent, about 3-4 minutes.

4. Add the minced garlic and cook for another minute until fragrant.

5. Add the chopped spinach to the skillet and cook until wilted, about 2-3 minutes.

6. Remove the skillet from heat and stir in the cooked quinoa, crumbled feta cheese, and dried oregano. Season with salt and pepper to taste.

7. Stuff each bell pepper with the spinach and feta mixture, packing it in tightly.

8. Place the stuffed bell peppers in a baking dish. Add a small amount of water (about 1/4 cup) to the bottom of the dish to help steam the peppers.

9. Cover the baking dish with foil and bake in the preheated oven for 30 minutes.

10. Remove the foil and bake for an additional 10-15 minutes, until the peppers are tender and slightly browned on top. Garnish with chopped fresh parsley before serving, if desired.

Nutritional Benefits:
- ***Bell Peppers:*** Rich in vitamins A and C, and antioxidants which are beneficial for immune health and reducing inflammation.
- ***Spinach:*** Provides iron, calcium, and folate, which are important for reproductive health.
- ***Quinoa:*** A complete protein that offers essential amino acids, fiber, and minerals.
- ***Feta Cheese:*** Adds a dose of calcium and protein, but should be used in moderation due to its sodium content.
- ***Olive Oil:*** Contains healthy monounsaturated fats that support hormone balance.

26. Chickpea Salad with Cucumber and Tomato

Ingredients:
- 1 can (15 oz) chickpeas, drained and rinsed
- 1 large cucumber, diced
- 2 cups cherry tomatoes, halved
- 1/4 red onion, finely chopped
- 1/4 cup fresh parsley, chopped
- 1/4 cup feta cheese, crumbled (optional)
- 2 tablespoons extra virgin olive oil
- 1 tablespoon lemon juice
- 1 tablespoon red wine vinegar
- 1 teaspoon dried oregano
- Salt and pepper to taste

Instructions:

1. In a large bowl, combine the chickpeas, diced cucumber, halved cherry tomatoes, chopped red onion, and chopped parsley.

2. In a small bowl, whisk together the olive oil, lemon juice, red wine vinegar, dried oregano, salt, and pepper until well combined.

3. Pour the dressing over the chickpea mixture and toss to coat all the ingredients evenly.

4. If using, gently fold in the crumbled feta cheese.

5. Adjust the seasoning with additional salt and pepper if needed.

6. Serve immediately or refrigerate for at least 30 minutes to allow the flavors to meld.

Nutritional Benefits:
- ***Chickpeas:*** Provide plant-based protein and fiber, helping to stabilize blood sugar levels and support digestive health.

- ***Cucumber***: Low in calories and high in water content, providing hydration and essential vitamins.

- ***Tomatoes:*** Rich in vitamins A and C, and lycopene, an antioxidant that helps reduce inflammation.

- ***Red Onion:*** Contains antioxidants and sulfur compounds that support heart health. A good source of vitamins K and C, and folate.

- ***Olive Oil:*** Contains healthy fats that help with hormone balance and anti-inflammatory properties.

- ***Lemon Juice and Red Wine Vinegar:*** Provide a fresh, tangy flavor and additional antioxidants.

27. Zucchini Noodles with Pesto and Cherry Tomatoes

Ingredients:
- 4 medium zucchinis, spiralized
- 1 cup cherry tomatoes, halved
- 2 tbsp olive oil
- Salt and pepper to taste
- For the Pesto:
  - 2 cups fresh basil
  - 1/4 cup pine nuts or walnuts
  - 1/2 cup grated Parmesan cheese
  - 2 cloves garlic
  - 1/2 cup extra virgin olive oil
  - Salt and pepper to taste
  - Juice of 1/2 lemon (optional)

Instructions:

1. Make the pesto by blending basil, nuts, Parmesan, garlic, and olive oil. Season and add lemon juice if desired.

2. Sauté zucchini noodles in olive oil until slightly softened, then add cherry tomatoes.

3. Toss noodles and tomatoes with pesto until coated.

4. Season with salt and pepper.

5. Garnish with toasted pine nuts if desired. Serve immediately.

Nutritional Benefits:

- Zucchini provides vitamins A and C.

- Basil offers antioxidants and anti-inflammatory properties.

- Pine nuts/walnuts provide healthy fats and protein.

- Parmesan adds flavor and calcium.

- Olive oil supports heart health and hormone balance.

- Cherry tomatoes are rich in vitamins and antioxidants.

This dish is both delicious and supports a PCOS fertility diet. Enjoy!

28. Salmon Salad with Spinach and Citrus Vinaigrette

Ingredients:
- 2 salmon fillets
- 4 cups fresh spinach
- 1 orange, segmented
- 1/4 cup sliced almonds
- 1/4 cup dried cranberries
- Salt and pepper

For the Citrus Vinaigrette:
- 2 tbsp orange juice
- 2 tbsp lemon juice
- 1 tbsp honey
- 2 tbsp olive oil
- Salt and pepper

Instructions:
1. Bake seasoned salmon fillets at 400°F (200°C) for 12-15 minutes until cooked.

2. Whisk together orange juice, lemon juice, honey, olive oil, salt, and pepper for the vinaigrette.

3. In a bowl, combine spinach, orange segments, almonds, and cranberries.

4. Flake cooked salmon into the salad.

5. Drizzle with citrus vinaigrette and toss gently.

6. Season with salt and pepper to taste.

Nutritional Benefits:
- Salmon provides omega-3 fatty acids for hormone balance.

- Spinach offers iron, calcium, and folate.

- Oranges provide vitamin C and antioxidants.

- Almonds are a source of healthy fats and protein.

- Dried cranberries add sweetness and antioxidants.

29. Brown Rice and Vegetable Stir-Fry

Ingredients:
- 2 tablespoons low-sodium soy sauce or tamari
- 1 tablespoon rice vinegar
- 1 teaspoon honey or maple syrup
- Optional toppings: sliced green onions, sesame seeds
- 2 cups cooked brown rice
- 2 cups mixed vegetables (such as bell peppers, broccoli, carrots, snap peas)
- 1 tablespoon sesame oil or olive oil
- 2 cloves garlic, minced
- 1 tablespoon grated ginger

Instructions:

1. Heat the sesame oil or olive oil in a large skillet or wok over medium heat.

2. Add minced garlic and grated ginger to the skillet and cook for 1-2 minutes until fragrant.

3. Add the mixed vegetables to the skillet and stir-fry for 5-7 minutes until they are crisp-tender.

4. In a small bowl, whisk together the soy sauce or tamari, rice vinegar, and honey or maple syrup.

5. Push the vegetables to one side of the skillet and add the cooked brown rice to the other side.

6. Pour the sauce over the rice and vegetables, and toss everything together until well combined.

7. Cook for an additional 2-3 minutes until heated through. Remove from heat and garnish with sliced green onions and sesame seeds if desired.

Nutritional Benefits:

- Brown Rice: Provides complex carbohydrates and fiber for stable energy levels.

- Mixed Vegetables: Rich in vitamins, minerals, and antioxidants that support overall health.

- Garlic and Ginger: Have anti-inflammatory properties and aid digestion.

- Soy Sauce or Tamari: Adds flavor and provides amino acids.

- Rice Vinegar: Adds tanginess and helps balance flavors. Adds sweetness and can be used in moderation for flavor.

30. Grilled Portobello Mushrooms with Quinoa

Ingredients:
- 4 large portobello mushrooms
- 1 cup quinoa, rinsed
- 2 cups vegetable broth or water
- 2 tbsp olive oil
- 2 cloves garlic, minced
- 1 tsp dried thyme
- Salt and pepper
- Optional toppings: chopped parsley, balsamic glaze

Instructions:

1. Cook quinoa in broth/water according to package instructions.

2. Preheat grill to medium-high heat.

3. Clean mushrooms, remove stems, and brush with olive oil mixture.

4. Grill mushrooms 4-5 minutes each side until tender.

5. Serve mushrooms over cooked quinoa.

6. Garnish with parsley and drizzle with balsamic glaze if desired.

Nutritional Benefits:

- Portobello Mushrooms: Low-cal, rich in nutrients.

- Quinoa: Complete protein source with fiber and essential nutrients.

- Olive Oil: Heart-healthy fats.

- Garlic and Thyme: Flavor with potential health benefits.

- Balsamic Glaze: Adds sweetness and acidity.

Enjoy this PCOS-friendly dish!

31. Baked Salmon with Asparagus

Ingredients:
- 4 salmon fillets
- 1 bunch asparagus, trimmed
- 2 tablespoons olive oil
- 2 cloves garlic, minced
- 1 lemon, thinly sliced
- Salt and pepper to taste
- Optional: Fresh herbs like dill or parsley for garnish

Instructions:
1. Preheat your oven to 400°F (200°C).

2. Place the salmon fillets on a baking sheet lined with parchment paper.

3. Arrange the trimmed asparagus around the salmon fillets on the baking sheet.

4. Drizzle the olive oil over the salmon and asparagus, then sprinkle minced garlic evenly over them. Season with salt and pepper to taste.

5. Place lemon slices on top of the salmon fillets.

6. Bake in the preheated oven for 12-15 minutes, or until the salmon is cooked through and flakes easily with a fork.

7. Remove from the oven and garnish with fresh herbs if desired.

8. Serve the baked salmon and asparagus hot, with additional lemon wedges if desired.

Nutritional Benefits:
- Salmon: Rich in omega-3 fatty acids which can help reduce inflammation and support hormone balance.

- Asparagus: Low in calories and high in fiber, folate, and vitamins A, C, and K.

- Olive Oil: Provides healthy fats that support heart health and hormone balance.

- Garlic: Adds flavor and has potential health benefits including anti-inflammatory properties.

- Lemon: Adds a fresh citrus flavor and is rich in vitamin C.

32. Quinoa-Stuffed Bell Peppers

Ingredients:
- 4 large bell peppers
- 1 cup quinoa
- 2 cups vegetable broth or water
- 1 tbsp olive oil
- 1 small onion, chopped
- 2 cloves garlic, minced
- 1 cup diced tomatoes
- 1 cup cooked black beans
- 1 tsp ground cumin
- 1 tsp chili powder
- Salt and pepper
- Optional toppings: cilantro, avocado slices, grated cheese

Instructions:
1. Preheat oven to 375°F (190°C).

2. Cook quinoa in broth/water as per package instructions.

3. Sauté onion and garlic in olive oil until softened.

4. Add tomatoes, black beans, cumin, chili powder, cooked quinoa, salt, and pepper. Cook briefly.

5. Stuff mixture into hollowed-out bell peppers.

6. Optionally, top with grated cheese.

7. Bake covered for 25-30 minutes until peppers are tender. Garnish with cilantro and avocado slices if desired.

Nutritional Benefits:
- Bell Peppers: Rich in vitamins and antioxidants.

- Quinoa: Complete protein source with fiber and minerals.

- Black Beans: Plant-based protein and fiber.

- Tomatoes: Vitamins and lycopene for inflammation reduction.

- Onion and Garlic: Flavor with potential health benefits.

- Avocado: Healthy fats and fiber for hormone regulation.

33. Grilled Chicken with Sweet Potatoes

Ingredients:
- 4 boneless, skinless chicken breasts
- 2 medium sweet potatoes, diced
- 2 tbsp olive oil
- 1 tsp paprika
- 1 tsp garlic powder
- 1 tsp dried thyme
- Salt and pepper
- Optional: Fresh herbs for garnish

Instructions:

1. Preheat grill to medium-high heat.

2. Toss sweet potatoes with 1 tbsp olive oil, paprika, garlic powder, thyme, salt, and pepper.
3. Grill sweet potatoes for 10-15 mins until tender.

4. Season chicken with remaining olive oil, salt, and pepper.

5. Grill chicken for 6-8 mins per side until cooked through.

6. Let chicken rest before serving.

7. Serve chicken with grilled sweet potatoes.

8. Garnish with fresh herbs if desired.

Nutritional Benefits:
- Chicken: Lean protein for muscle health.

- Sweet Potatoes: Complex carbs, fiber, vitamins A and C.

- Olive Oil: Heart-healthy fats and antioxidants.

- Paprika, Garlic Powder, Thyme: Flavor without added calories.

- Fresh Herbs: Flavor and potential health benefits.

Enjoy this PCOS-friendly Grilled Chicken with Sweet Potatoes!

34. Lentil and Vegetable Stew

Ingredients:
- 1 cup dried green or brown lentils, rinsed
- 4 cups vegetable broth or water
- 1 tbsp olive oil
- 1 onion, diced
- 2 cloves garlic, minced
- 2 carrots, diced
- 2 celery stalks, diced
- 1 bell pepper, diced
- 1 can (14 oz) diced tomatoes
- 2 cups chopped spinach or kale
- 1 tsp dried thyme
- 1 tsp dried oregano
- Salt and pepper
- Optional toppings: chopped parsley, lemon wedges

Instructions:

1. Sauté onion and garlic in olive oil until softened.

2. Add carrots, celery, bell pepper, lentils, tomatoes, thyme, oregano, and broth. Simmer for 20-25 mins.

3. Add spinach or kale and cook for 5 more mins.

4. Season with salt and pepper. Serve hot, garnished with parsley and lemon wedges if desired.

Nutritional Benefits:

- Lentils: Fiber and plant-based protein.

- Vegetables: Vitamins, minerals, antioxidants.

- Tomatoes: Vitamin C, lycopene for inflammation.

- Leafy Greens: Additional fiber, vitamins, minerals.

- Herbs: Flavor and potential health benefits.

Enjoy this PCOS-friendly Lentil and Vegetable Stew!

35. Shrimp and Vegetable Skewers

Ingredients:
- 1 lb large shrimp, peeled and deveined
- 2 zucchinis, sliced
- 1 bell pepper, cut into chunks
- 1 red onion, cut into chunks
- 1 lemon, sliced
- 2 tbsp olive oil
- 2 cloves garlic, minced
- 1 tsp dried oregano
- Salt and pepper
- Optional: Fresh herbs for garnish

Instructions:

1. Soak wooden skewers in water.

2. Combine shrimp, vegetables, and lemon slices in a bowl.

3. Whisk olive oil, garlic, oregano, salt, and pepper for marinade. Pour over shrimp and vegetables, marinate for 15 minutes.

4. Preheat grill to medium-high heat.

5. Thread shrimp and vegetables onto skewers.

6. Grill skewers for 3-4 minutes per side until shrimp are pink and veggies are tender.

7. Garnish with fresh herbs if desired, serve hot.

Enjoy these PCOS-friendly Shrimp and Vegetable Skewers!

36. Turkey Meatballs with Zucchini Noodles

Ingredients:
- 1 lb ground turkey
- 1 egg
- 1/4 cup almond flour
- 1/4 cup grated Parmesan cheese
- 2 cloves garlic, minced
- 1 tsp dried oregano
- 1/2 tsp salt
- 1/4 tsp black pepper
- 3 medium zucchinis, spiralized into noodles
- 1 cup marinara sauce

Instructions:

1. In a large bowl, combine the ground turkey, egg, almond flour, Parmesan, garlic, oregano, salt, and pepper. Mix well until fully incorporated.

2. Roll the mixture into 1-inch meatballs and place them on a baking sheet lined with parchment paper.

3. Bake the meatballs at 400°F for 18-20 minutes, or until cooked through.

4. While the meatballs are baking, spiralize the zucchinis into noodles.

5. In a large skillet, heat the marinara sauce over medium heat. Add the zucchini noodles and toss to coat.

6. Serve the zucchini noodles topped with the baked turkey meatballs.

This recipe is a great option for a PCOS fertility diet as it is high in protein from the turkey, low in carbs from the zucchini noodles, and contains healthy fats from the almond flour and Parmesan cheese. The vegetables also provide important nutrients and fiber. Enjoy!

37. Baked Cod with Lemon and Herbs

Ingredients:
- 1 lb cod fillets
- 2 tbsp olive oil
- 2 tbsp fresh lemon juice
- 2 cloves garlic, minced
- 2 tbsp chopped fresh parsley
- 1 tbsp chopped fresh dill
- 1 tsp dried oregano
- 1/2 tsp salt
- 1/4 tsp black pepper

Instructions:

1. Preheat your oven to 400°F (200°C).

2. In a small bowl, mix together the olive oil, lemon juice, garlic, parsley, dill, oregano, salt, and pepper.

3. Place the cod fillets in a baking dish and pour the lemon-herb mixture over the top, making sure to evenly coat the fish.

4. Bake the cod for 15-20 minutes, or until it flakes easily with a fork and is opaque throughout.

5. Serve the baked cod immediately, garnished with additional fresh herbs if desired.

This recipe is an excellent choice for a PCOS fertility diet as cod is a lean, high-protein fish that is rich in omega-3 fatty acids, which can help reduce inflammation and support fertility. The lemon and herbs add flavor without the need for additional salt or unhealthy fats. Pair this dish with a side of roasted vegetables or a fresh salad for a complete and nutritious meal.

38. Vegetarian Chili with Beans and Lentils

Ingredients:
- 1 tbsp olive oil
- 1 onion, diced
- 3 cloves garlic, minced
- 1 red bell pepper, diced
- 1 cup uncooked lentils, rinsed
- 1 (15 oz) can black beans, drained and rinsed
- 1 (15 oz) can kidney beans, drained and rinsed
- 1 (28 oz) can diced tomatoes
- 2 cups vegetable broth
- 2 tbsp chili powder
- 1 tsp ground cumin
- 1 tsp dried oregano
- 1/2 tsp smoked paprika
- 1/4 tsp cayenne pepper (optional, for heat)
- Salt and black pepper to taste

Instructions:

1. In a large pot or Dutch oven, heat the olive oil over medium heat. Add the onion and sauté for 5 minutes until translucent.

2. Add the garlic and bell pepper, and sauté for an additional 2-3 minutes.

3. Stir in the lentils, black beans, kidney beans, diced tomatoes, and vegetable broth. Season with chili powder, cumin, oregano, smoked paprika, and cayenne (if using).

4. Bring the mixture to a boil, then reduce heat and let it simmer for 25-30 minutes, or until the lentils are tender.

5. Season with salt and black pepper to taste.

6. Serve the chili hot, garnished with avocado, cilantro, or other desired toppings.

This vegetarian chili is an excellent choice for a PCOS fertility diet as it is high in fiber, protein, and complex carbohydrates from the beans and lentils. The vegetables and spices also provide important nutrients and antioxidants. Enjoy this hearty and nutritious meal!

39. Grilled Tofu with Brown Rice

Ingredients:
- 1 block (14 oz) extra-firm tofu, pressed and cut into 1/2-inch thick slices
- 2 tbsp low-sodium soy sauce or tamari
- 1 tbsp sesame oil
- 1 tbsp rice vinegar
- 1 tsp honey
- 1 tsp grated ginger
- 1 clove garlic, minced
- 1/4 tsp red pepper flakes (optional)
- 2 cups cooked brown rice
- 2 cups steamed broccoli or other vegetables

Instructions:

1. In a shallow dish, whisk together the soy sauce, sesame oil, rice vinegar, honey, ginger, garlic, and red pepper flakes (if using).

2. Add the tofu slices to the marinade and gently toss to coat. Let the tofu marinate for at least 30 minutes, flipping the slices halfway through.

3. Preheat a grill or grill pan over medium-high heat. Carefully place the marinated tofu slices on the grill and cook for 3-4 minutes per side, or until grill marks appear and the tofu is lightly charred.

4. Serve the grilled tofu over the cooked brown rice, accompanied by the steamed broccoli or other vegetables.

This dish is an excellent choice for a PCOS fertility diet as it is high in protein from the tofu, complex carbohydrates from the brown rice, and fiber and nutrients from the vegetables. The marinade adds flavor without the need for excessive salt or unhealthy fats. Feel free to adjust the vegetables or add other PCOS-friendly ingredients to suit your preferences.

40. Eggplant Parmesan with Whole Wheat Pasta

Ingredients:
- 1 large eggplant, sliced into 1/2-inch thick rounds
- 1 cup whole wheat breadcrumbs
- 1/2 cup grated Parmesan cheese
- 2 eggs, beaten
- 2 tbsp olive oil
- 1 (24 oz) jar marinara sauce
- 1 cup shredded part-skim mozzarella cheese
- 8 oz whole wheat pasta

Instructions:

1. Preheat your oven to 375°F (190°C). Line a baking sheet with parchment paper.

2. In a shallow dish, combine the breadcrumbs and Parmesan cheese. In a separate shallow dish, place the beaten eggs.

3. Dip the eggplant slices into the egg, then coat them in the breadcrumb mixture, pressing gently to adhere.

4. Arrange the breaded eggplant slices on the prepared baking sheet. Drizzle with the olive oil.

5. Bake the eggplant for 20-25 minutes, flipping halfway, until golden brown and tender.

6. In a baking dish, spread a thin layer of marinara sauce. Arrange the baked eggplant slices in a single layer, then top with the remaining marinara sauce and the shredded mozzarella cheese.

7. Bake the eggplant Parmesan for an additional 15-20 minutes, or until the cheese is melted and bubbly.

8. Meanwhile, cook the whole wheat pasta according to the package instructions. Drain and serve the eggplant Parmesan over the cooked pasta.

This eggplant Parmesan dish is a great option for a PCOS fertility diet as it is low in carbs, high in fiber, and contains healthy fats from the olive oil and cheese. The whole wheat pasta provides complex carbohydrates to help balance blood sugar levels. Enjoy this nutritious and delicious meal!

41. Dark Chocolate-Dipped Strawberries

Ingredients:
- 1 lb fresh strawberries, washed and dried thoroughly
- 4 oz dark chocolate (at least 70% cacao), chopped
- 1 tbsp coconut oil (or other neutral-flavored oil)

Instructions:

1. Line a baking sheet with parchment paper or a silicone mat.

2. In a double boiler or a heatproof bowl set over a saucepan of simmering water, melt the dark chocolate and coconut oil, stirring occasionally until smooth.

3. Carefully dip each strawberry into the melted chocolate, coating about three-quarters of the berry. Gently shake off any excess chocolate.

4. Place the chocolate-dipped strawberries on the prepared baking sheet, making sure they are not touching each other.

5. Refrigerate the strawberries for at least 30 minutes, or until the chocolate has set.

6. Serve the dark chocolate-dipped strawberries chilled.

These dark chocolate-dipped strawberries are a great option for a PCOS fertility diet because they are low in carbs, high in fiber, and contain antioxidants from the dark chocolate. The combination of the sweet, juicy strawberries and the rich, dark chocolate is both delicious and satisfying.

Remember to choose a high-quality dark chocolate with a cacao content of at least 70% to maximize the health benefits. Enjoy these treats in moderation as part of a balanced PCOS-friendly diet.

42. Almond Flour Cookies

Ingredients:
- 2 cups almond flour
- 1/4 cup coconut oil, melted
- 1/4 cup honey or maple syrup
- 1 egg
- 1 tsp vanilla extract
- 1/4 tsp baking soda
- 1/4 tsp salt

Instructions:

1. Preheat oven to 350°F. Line a baking sheet with parchment paper.

2. In a medium bowl, whisk together the almond flour, baking soda, and salt.

3. In a separate bowl, whisk together the melted coconut oil, honey/maple syrup, egg, and vanilla.

4. Stir the wet ingredients into the dry ingredients until a dough forms.

5. Scoop tablespoon-sized balls of dough onto the prepared baking sheet, spacing them a few inches apart.

6. Bake for 10-12 minutes, until lightly golden on the edges.

7. Allow the cookies to cool on the baking sheet for 5 minutes before transferring to a wire rack to cool completely.

These almond flour cookies are grain-free, gluten-free, and sweetened with natural honey or maple syrup, making them a good option for a PCOS fertility diet. The almond flour provides healthy fats and protein. Enjoy!

43. Coconut Yogurt with Mango

Ingredients:
- 1 cup full-fat coconut yogurt
- 1 cup diced fresh mango
- 1 tbsp unsweetened shredded coconut (optional)
- 1 tsp honey or maple syrup (optional)

Instructions:

1. Spoon the coconut yogurt into a serving bowl or individual bowls.

2. Top the yogurt with the diced mango.

3. Sprinkle the unsweetened shredded coconut over the top, if using.

4. Drizzle with a small amount of honey or maple syrup, if desired.

This coconut yogurt with mango makes a delicious and nutritious snack or light breakfast. The coconut yogurt provides healthy fats and probiotics, while the mango adds natural sweetness and fiber. This dish is gluten-free, dairy-free, and can be made low in added sugars by using minimal or no honey/maple syrup.

The healthy fats, fiber, and low-glycemic nature of this recipe make it a great option for a PCOS fertility diet. The nutrients can help support hormone balance and reproductive health. Enjoy this refreshing and nourishing coconut yogurt and mango treat!

44. Chia Seed Pudding with Coconut Milk

Ingredients:
- 1/4 cup chia seeds
- 1 cup unsweetened coconut milk
- 1 tbsp honey or maple syrup (optional)
- 1/2 tsp vanilla extract
- 1/4 tsp ground cinnamon
- Fresh berries, nuts, or shredded coconut for topping (optional)

Instructions:
1. In a medium bowl, whisk together the chia seeds, coconut milk, honey/maple syrup (if using), vanilla, and cinnamon until well combined.

2. Cover the bowl and refrigerate for at least 2 hours, or overnight, stirring occasionally, until the chia seeds have thickened the mixture into a pudding-like consistency.

3. Divide the chia seed pudding into individual serving bowls or jars.

4. Top with fresh berries, chopped nuts, or shredded coconut, if desired.

This chia seed pudding is a nutritious and satisfying snack or breakfast option. The chia seeds provide fiber, protein, and omega-3 fatty acids, while the coconut milk offers healthy fats. The optional honey or maple syrup adds a touch of sweetness.

This recipe is gluten-free, dairy-free, and can be made low in added sugars by using minimal or no honey/maple syrup. The healthy fats, fiber, and low-glycemic nature of the ingredients make this chia seed pudding a great choice for a PCOS fertility diet. Enjoy!

45. Baked Apples with Cinnamon and Walnuts

Ingredients:
- 4 medium-sized apples (such as Honeycrisp or Gala)
- 1/4 cup chopped walnuts
- 2 tbsp coconut oil, melted
- 1 tbsp honey or maple syrup (optional)
- 1 tsp ground cinnamon
- 1/4 tsp ground nutmeg

Instructions:
1. Preheat the oven to 375°F. Lightly grease a baking dish or line it with parchment paper.

2. Core the apples, leaving the bottom intact so they can stand upright. Use a paring knife or melon baller to scoop out the core, creating a well in the center of each apple.

3. In a small bowl, mix together the chopped walnuts, melted coconut oil, honey/maple syrup (if using), cinnamon, and nutmeg.

4. Spoon the walnut mixture evenly into the center of each apple.

5. Place the stuffed apples in the prepared baking dish.

6. Bake for 30-40 minutes, or until the apples are tender when pierced with a fork.

7. Serve the baked apples warm, with any juices from the baking dish spooned over the top.

These baked apples make a delicious and nutritious dessert or snack. The walnuts provide healthy fats and protein, while the apples and spices offer fiber and antioxidants. This recipe is gluten-free, dairy-free, and can be made low in added sugars by using minimal or no honey/maple syrup.

The combination of fiber, healthy fats, and low-glycemic ingredients makes this dish a great choice for a PCOS fertility diet. Enjoy these cozy, comforting baked apples!

46. Fresh Berry Compote with Greek Yogurt

Ingredients:
- 2 cups mixed fresh berries (such as strawberries, blueberries, raspberries)
- 1 tbsp honey or maple syrup (optional)
- 1 tsp lemon juice
- 1 cup plain full-fat Greek yogurt

Instructions:

1. In a medium saucepan, combine the mixed berries, honey/maple syrup (if using), and lemon juice.

2. Cook over medium heat, stirring occasionally, until the berries release their juices and the mixture thickens slightly, about 10-15 minutes.

3. Remove the berry compote from heat and let it cool slightly.

4. Divide the Greek yogurt evenly among serving bowls or cups.

5. Top the yogurt with the warm berry compote.

This fresh berry compote with Greek yogurt makes a delicious and nutritious breakfast, snack, or dessert. The berries provide antioxidants, fiber, and natural sweetness, while the Greek yogurt offers protein and probiotics.

This recipe is gluten-free, and can be made dairy-free by using a non-dairy yogurt alternative. The minimal added sweetener (honey or maple syrup) makes it a suitable option for a PCOS fertility diet. The combination of protein, fiber, and low-glycemic ingredients can help support hormone balance and reproductive health.

Enjoy this refreshing and nourishing berry and yogurt treat!

47. Avocado Chocolate Mousse

Ingredients:
- 2 ripe avocados, pitted and flesh scooped out
- 1/4 cup unsweetened cocoa powder
- 1/4 cup honey or maple syrup
- 1/4 cup unsweetened almond milk
- 1 tsp vanilla extract
- 1/4 tsp sea salt

Instructions:
1. In a food processor or high-powered blender, combine the avocado flesh, cocoa powder, honey/maple syrup, almond milk, vanilla, and salt. Blend until smooth and creamy, scraping down the sides as needed.

2. Taste and adjust sweetener or other ingredients as desired.

3. Transfer the chocolate mousse to individual serving bowls or cups.

4. Refrigerate for at least 30 minutes before serving to allow the mousse to set.

5. Top with fresh berries, chopped nuts, or a sprinkle of unsweetened cocoa powder, if desired.

This avocado chocolate mousse is a rich and decadent treat that is also nutritious. The avocado provides healthy fats, fiber, and creaminess, while the cocoa powder and sweetener offer a chocolatey flavor. The minimal added sweetener makes this recipe suitable for a PCOS fertility diet.

This dessert is gluten-free, dairy-free, and can be made vegan by using maple syrup instead of honey. The healthy fats, fiber, and low-glycemic nature of the ingredients make this avocado chocolate mousse a great option for supporting hormone balance and reproductive health.

Enjoy this indulgent yet nourishing chocolate mousse!

48. Almond Butter Brownies

Ingredients:
- 1 cup almond butter
- 1/2 cup unsweetened cocoa powder
- 1/4 cup honey or maple syrup
- 2 eggs
- 1 tsp vanilla extract
- 1/4 tsp sea salt

Instructions:
1. Preheat the oven to 350°F. Grease an 8x8-inch baking pan with coconut oil or line it with parchment paper.

2. In a medium bowl, whisk together the almond butter, cocoa powder, honey/maple syrup, eggs, vanilla, and salt until well combined.

3. Spread the brownie batter evenly into the prepared baking pan.

4. Bake for 18-22 minutes, or until the edges are set and a toothpick inserted in the center comes out clean.

5. Allow the brownies to cool completely in the pan before cutting into squares.

6. Serve the almond butter brownies at room temperature or chilled.

These almond butter brownies are a delicious and nutritious treat that are perfect for a PCOS fertility diet. The almond butter provides healthy fats and protein, while the cocoa powder and minimal sweetener offer a rich chocolate flavor.

This recipe is gluten-free, grain-free, and can be made dairy-free. The low-glycemic nature of the ingredients makes these brownies a great option for supporting hormone balance and reproductive health.

Enjoy these fudgy and satisfying almond butter brownies as a guilt-free indulgence!

49. Frozen Banana Bites with Dark Chocolate

Ingredients:
- 2 ripe bananas, peeled and sliced into 1/2-inch thick rounds
- 1/2 cup dark chocolate chips or chopped dark chocolate
- 1 tbsp coconut oil

Instructions:
1. Line a baking sheet or plate with parchment paper.

2. Arrange the banana slices in a single layer on the prepared surface.

3. In a small microwave-safe bowl, combine the dark chocolate chips and coconut oil. Microwave in 30-second intervals, stirring in between, until the chocolate is melted and smooth.

4. Using a fork or spoon, drizzle or dip the banana slices into the melted chocolate, coating them partially or fully.

5. Place the chocolate-dipped banana bites back on the parchment-lined surface and freeze for at least 2 hours, or until firm.

6. Once frozen, transfer the banana bites to an airtight container or resealable bag and store in the freezer until ready to serve.

These frozen banana bites with dark chocolate make a delicious and healthy snack or dessert. The bananas provide natural sweetness and potassium, while the dark chocolate offers antioxidants and a rich, indulgent flavor.

This recipe is gluten-free, dairy-free, and can be made with minimal added sweetener, making it a great option for a PCOS fertility diet. The healthy fats from the coconut oil and dark chocolate, along with the fiber and low-glycemic nature of the ingredients, can help support hormone balance and reproductive health.

Enjoy these frozen banana bites as a refreshing and satisfying treat!

50. Date and Nut Energy Balls

Ingredients:
- 1 cup pitted Medjool dates
- 1/2 cup raw almonds
- 1/2 cup raw walnuts
- 2 tbsp unsweetened shredded coconut
- 1 tbsp chia seeds
- 1 tsp vanilla extract
- 1/4 tsp ground cinnamon
- Pinch of sea salt

Instructions:

1. In a food processor, combine the pitted dates, almonds, walnuts, shredded coconut, chia seeds, vanilla, cinnamon, and salt. Pulse until the mixture is finely chopped and starts to stick together.

2. Scoop the date and nut mixture by the tablespoonful and roll into small balls with your hands.

3. Place the energy balls on a parchment-lined baking sheet or plate.

4. Refrigerate the energy balls for at least 30 minutes to allow them to firm up.

5. Store the energy balls in an airtight container in the refrigerator for up to 1 week.

These date and nut energy balls are a nutrient-dense and satisfying snack or treat. The dates provide natural sweetness, while the nuts and seeds offer healthy fats, protein, and fiber. The minimal ingredients make this recipe suitable for a PCOS fertility diet.

This recipe is gluten-free, dairy-free, and can be made vegan. The combination of fiber, healthy fats, and low-glycemic ingredients can help support hormone balance and reproductive health.

Enjoy these easy-to-make, portable energy balls as a nourishing on-the-go option!

51. Vegetable and Tofu Stir-Fry

Ingredients:
- 1 block (14 oz) firm or extra-firm tofu, cubed
- 2 tbsp coconut oil or avocado oil
- 1 cup sliced mushrooms
- 1 cup broccoli florets
- 1 cup sliced bell peppers
- 1 cup snow peas or snap peas
- 3 cloves garlic, minced
- 1 tbsp grated fresh ginger
- 2 tbsp low-sodium tamari or coconut aminos
- 1 tsp sesame oil
- 1/4 tsp red pepper flakes (optional)
- Salt and black pepper to taste
- Chopped green onions or cilantro for garnish (optional)

Instructions:

1. In a large skillet or wok, heat the coconut or avocado oil over medium-high heat.

2. Add the cubed tofu and cook, stirring occasionally, until lightly browned on all sides, about 5-7 minutes. Transfer the tofu to a plate.

3. In the same skillet, add the mushrooms, broccoli, bell peppers, and snow peas. Stir-fry for 3-5 minutes, until the vegetables are crisp-tender.

4. Add the garlic and ginger and cook for 1 minute, until fragrant.

5. Return the tofu to the skillet and add the tamari/coconut aminos, sesame oil, and red pepper flakes (if using). Toss everything together and cook for 2-3 minutes, until heated through.

6. Season with salt and black pepper to taste.

7. Serve the vegetable and tofu stir-fry over steamed quinoa or cauliflower rice. Garnish with chopped green onions or cilantro, if desired.

This vegetable and tofu stir-fry is a nutritious and flavorful dish that is suitable for a PCOS fertility diet. The tofu provides plant-based protein, while the vegetables offer fiber, vitamins, and minerals. The minimal use of oil and low-sodium soy sauce or coconut aminos keeps the dish light and low in added sugars.

This recipe is gluten-free, dairy-free, and can be made vegan. The combination of protein, fiber, and low-glycemic ingredients can help support hormone balance and reproductive health.

52. Spaghetti Squash with Marinara Sauce

Ingredients:
- 1 medium spaghetti squash, halved lengthwise and seeds removed
- 1 tbsp olive oil
- 1 onion, diced
- 3 cloves garlic, minced
- 1 (28 oz) can diced tomatoes
- 2 tbsp tomato paste
- 1 tsp dried oregano
- 1/2 tsp dried basil
- 1/4 tsp red pepper flakes (optional)
- Salt and black pepper to taste
- Chopped fresh basil for garnish (optional)

Instructions:
1. Preheat the oven to 400°F. Place the spaghetti squash halves cut-side down on a baking sheet. Bake for 40-50 minutes, or until the squash is tender and easily shreds with a fork.

2. In a large skillet, heat the olive oil over medium heat. Add the diced onion and sauté for 5-7 minutes, until translucent.

3. Add the minced garlic and cook for 1 minute, until fragrant.

4. Stir in the diced tomatoes, tomato paste, oregano, basil, and red pepper flakes (if using). Season with salt and black pepper to taste.

5. Simmer the marinara sauce for 10-15 minutes, stirring occasionally, until thickened.

6. Use a fork to shred the cooked spaghetti squash into strands. Transfer the squash strands to serving plates or bowls.

7. Top the spaghetti squash with the warm marinara sauce and garnish with chopped fresh basil, if desired.

This spaghetti squash with marinara sauce is a delicious and nutritious alternative to traditional pasta dishes. The spaghetti squash provides fiber and nutrients, while the homemade marinara sauce is low in added sugars.

This recipe is gluten-free, dairy-free, and suitable for a PCOS fertility diet. The fiber, low-glycemic nature, and nutrient-dense ingredients can help support hormone balance and reproductive health.

53. Chicken and Vegetable Kabobs

Ingredients:
- 1 lb boneless, skinless chicken breasts, cut into 1-inch cubes
- 1 red bell pepper, cut into 1-inch pieces
- 1 zucchini, cut into 1-inch slices
- 1 red onion, cut into 1-inch pieces
- 8 oz mushrooms, halved
- 2 tbsp olive oil
- 2 tbsp lemon juice
- 1 tsp dried oregano
- 1 tsp dried basil
- 1/2 tsp garlic powder
- Salt and black pepper to taste
- Wooden or metal skewers

Instructions:

1. In a large bowl, combine the cubed chicken, bell pepper, zucchini, red onion, and mushrooms.

2. In a small bowl, whisk together the olive oil, lemon juice, oregano, basil, garlic powder, salt, and black pepper.

3. Pour the marinade over the chicken and vegetables and toss to coat everything evenly.

4. Thread the marinated chicken and vegetables onto the skewers, alternating the ingredients.

5. Preheat your grill or grill pan to medium-high heat.

6. Grill the kabobs for 12-15 minutes, turning occasionally, until the chicken is cooked through and the vegetables are tender.

7. Serve the chicken and vegetable kabobs immediately, with any remaining marinade drizzled over the top.

These chicken and vegetable kabobs are a great option for a PCOS fertility diet. The lean chicken provides protein, while the variety of vegetables offer fiber, vitamins, and minerals. The minimal use of oil and no added sugars keep the dish light and nutritious.

This recipe is gluten-free, dairy-free, and can be made low-carb by using more vegetables and less chicken. The combination of protein, fiber, and low-glycemic ingredients can help support hormone balance and reproductive health.

54. Cauliflower Rice with Herbs and Spices

Ingredients:
- 1 head of cauliflower, cut into florets
- 2 tbsp olive oil
- 2 cloves garlic, minced
- 1 tsp ground cumin
- 1 tsp dried oregano
- 1/2 tsp ground coriander
- 1/4 tsp ground turmeric
- 1/4 tsp red pepper flakes (optional)
- Salt and black pepper to taste
- Chopped fresh parsley or cilantro for garnish (optional)

Instructions:
1. In a food processor, pulse the cauliflower florets in batches until they are broken down into small, rice-like pieces.

2. In a large skillet or wok, heat the olive oil over medium heat. Add the minced garlic and sauté for 1 minute, until fragrant.

3. Add the riced cauliflower, cumin, oregano, coriander, turmeric, and red pepper flakes (if using). Stir to combine.

4. Cook the cauliflower rice, stirring occasionally, for 5-7 minutes, until it's tender and heated through.

5. Season the cauliflower rice with salt and black pepper to taste.

6. Transfer the cauliflower rice to a serving bowl and garnish with chopped fresh parsley or cilantro, if desired.

This cauliflower rice with herbs and spices is a delicious and nutritious alternative to traditional rice. Cauliflower is low in carbs and high in fiber, making it a great option for a PCOS fertility diet.

The combination of aromatic spices and herbs adds flavor without the need for added sugars or unhealthy fats. This recipe is gluten-free, dairy-free, and can be made vegan.

The fiber, low-glycemic nature, and nutrient-dense ingredients in this cauliflower rice dish can help support hormone balance and reproductive health. Enjoy it as a side dish or as a base for other PCOS-friendly meals.

55. Baked Chicken with Brussels Sprouts

Ingredients:
- 1 lb boneless, skinless chicken breasts, cut into 1-inch cubes
- 1 lb Brussels sprouts, trimmed and halved
- 2 tbsp olive oil
- 2 cloves garlic, minced
- 1 tsp dried thyme
- 1/2 tsp paprika
- Salt and black pepper to taste

Instructions:
1. Preheat the oven to 400°F. Line a large baking sheet with parchment paper.

2. In a large bowl, toss the cubed chicken, Brussels sprouts, olive oil, garlic, thyme, paprika, salt, and black pepper until everything is evenly coated.

3. Spread the chicken and Brussels sprouts mixture in a single layer on the prepared baking sheet.

4. Bake for 20-25 minutes, stirring halfway, until the chicken is cooked through and the Brussels sprouts are tender and lightly browned.

5. Serve the baked chicken and Brussels sprouts immediately, garnished with additional fresh thyme or parsley, if desired.

This baked chicken and Brussels sprouts dish is a simple and nutritious meal that is perfect for a PCOS fertility diet. The lean chicken provides protein, while the Brussels sprouts offer fiber, vitamins, and minerals.

The minimal use of oil and no added sugars keep this recipe light and low in carbs. This dish is gluten-free, dairy-free, and can be made low-carb by adjusting the portion sizes.

The combination of protein, fiber, and low-glycemic ingredients in this recipe can help support hormone balance and reproductive health. Enjoy this flavorful and satisfying baked chicken and Brussels sprouts dish!

56. Sweet Potato and Black Bean Tacos

Ingredients:
- 2 medium sweet potatoes, peeled and diced
- 1 tbsp olive oil
- 1 tsp ground cumin
- 1/2 tsp chili powder
- Salt and black pepper to taste
- 1 (15 oz) can black beans, rinsed and drained
- 1 avocado, diced
- 1/4 cup chopped red onion
- 2 tbsp chopped fresh cilantro
- 8-10 small corn tortillas or lettuce wraps
- Lime wedges for serving

Instructions:
1. Preheat the oven to 400°F. Line a baking sheet with parchment paper.

2. In a large bowl, toss the diced sweet potatoes with the olive oil, cumin, chili powder, salt, and black pepper until evenly coated.

3. Spread the seasoned sweet potato cubes in a single layer on the prepared baking sheet.

4. Roast the sweet potatoes for 20-25 minutes, stirring halfway, until they are tender and lightly browned.

5. In a medium bowl, combine the roasted sweet potatoes, black beans, diced avocado, red onion, and chopped cilantro. Gently mix to incorporate. Warm the corn tortillas or prepare the lettuce wraps according to package instructions.

7. Spoon the sweet potato and black bean mixture into the tortillas or lettuce wraps. Serve the tacos with lime wedges for squeezing over the top.

These sweet potato and black bean tacos are a delicious and nutritious option for a PCOS fertility diet. The sweet potatoes provide complex carbs, fiber, and vitamins, while the black beans offer protein and fiber. The avocado and minimal use of oil keep the dish heart-healthy.

This recipe is gluten-free, dairy-free, and can be made vegan by omitting the cheese or using a non-dairy alternative. The combination of fiber, protein, and low-glycemic ingredients can help support hormone balance and reproductive health.

57. Greek Salad with Feta and Olives

Ingredients:
- 6 cups chopped romaine lettuce
- 1 cup cherry tomatoes, halved
- 1 cucumber, diced
- 1/2 red onion, thinly sliced
- 1/2 cup pitted kalamata olives, halved
- 1/4 cup crumbled feta cheese
- 2 tbsp olive oil
- 1 tbsp red wine vinegar
- 1 tsp dried oregano
- 1 clove garlic, minced
- Salt and black pepper to taste

Instructions:

1. In a large salad bowl, combine the chopped romaine lettuce, cherry tomatoes, diced cucumber, sliced red onion, and halved kalamata olives.

2. Sprinkle the crumbled feta cheese over the top of the salad.

3. In a small bowl, whisk together the olive oil, red wine vinegar, dried oregano, and minced garlic. Season with salt and black pepper to taste.

4. Drizzle the dressing over the salad and gently toss to coat everything evenly.

5. Serve the Greek salad immediately, or refrigerate until ready to serve.

This Greek salad is a refreshing and nutritious option for a PCOS fertility diet. The leafy greens, vegetables, and olives provide fiber, vitamins, and antioxidants. The feta cheese adds a creamy, tangy flavor and a source of protein.

The simple olive oil and vinegar dressing keeps the salad light and low in added sugars. This recipe is gluten-free and can be made dairy-free by omitting the feta cheese.

The combination of fiber, healthy fats, and low-glycemic ingredients in this Greek salad can help support hormone balance and reproductive health. Enjoy this flavorful and satisfying salad as a main dish or a side.

58. Roasted Vegetable Medley

Ingredients:
- 1 medium zucchini, cut into 1-inch pieces
- 1 medium yellow squash, cut into 1-inch pieces
- 1 red bell pepper, cut into 1-inch pieces
- 1 cup Brussels sprouts, trimmed and halved
- 1 cup cauliflower florets
- 1 red onion, cut into 1-inch pieces
- 2 tbsp olive oil
- 1 tsp dried thyme
- 1 tsp dried oregano
- 1/2 tsp garlic powder
- Salt and black pepper to taste
- Chopped fresh parsley for garnish (optional)

Instructions:
1. Preheat the oven to 400°F. Line a large baking sheet with parchment paper.

2. In a large bowl, combine the zucchini, yellow squash, bell pepper, Brussels sprouts, cauliflower, and red onion.

3. Drizzle the vegetables with the olive oil and sprinkle with the dried thyme, oregano, garlic powder, salt, and black pepper. Toss to coat everything evenly.

4. Spread the seasoned vegetables in a single layer on the prepared baking sheet.

5. Roast the vegetables for 25-30 minutes, stirring halfway, until they are tender and lightly browned.

6. Transfer the roasted vegetable medley to a serving dish and garnish with chopped fresh parsley, if desired.

This roasted vegetable medley is a simple and nutritious side dish that is perfect for a PCOS fertility diet. The variety of vegetables provides a range of fiber, vitamins, minerals, and antioxidants.

The recipe is gluten-free, dairy-free, and vegan, making it suitable for various dietary needs. The minimal use of oil and no added sugars keep the dish light and low in carbs.

The combination of fiber, low-glycemic ingredients, and nutrient-dense vegetables in this roasted medley can help support hormone balance and reproductive health. Enjoy this flavorful and colorful side dish!

59. Stuffed Zucchini Boats

Ingredients:
- 4 medium zucchini, halved lengthwise
- 1 lb ground turkey or chicken
- 1 cup diced tomatoes
- 1/2 cup cooked quinoa
- 1/4 cup chopped fresh basil
- 2 cloves garlic, minced
- 1 tsp dried oregano
- 1/4 tsp red pepper flakes (optional)
- Salt and black pepper to taste
- 1/4 cup shredded mozzarella cheese (optional)

Instructions:
1. Preheat the oven to 375°F. Lightly grease a baking dish or line it with parchment paper.

2. Using a spoon or melon baller, scoop out the flesh from the center of each zucchini half, leaving a 1/4-inch border. Chop the scooped-out zucchini flesh.

3. In a large skillet, cook the ground turkey or chicken over medium heat, breaking it up with a spatula, until no longer pink, about 5-7 minutes.

4. Add the chopped zucchini flesh, diced tomatoes, cooked quinoa, fresh basil, garlic, oregano, and red pepper flakes (if using) to the skillet. Season with salt and black pepper to taste. Stir to combine.

5. Spoon the turkey/chicken and vegetable mixture evenly into the zucchini boats, pressing it down gently.

6. Place the stuffed zucchini boats in the prepared baking dish.

7. Bake for 20-25 minutes, or until the zucchini is tender. If using mozzarella cheese, sprinkle it over the top during the last 5 minutes of baking. Serve the stuffed zucchini boats warm.

These stuffed zucchini boats are a delicious and nutritious main dish that is perfect for a PCOS fertility diet. The zucchini provides fiber and nutrients, while the ground turkey or chicken offers protein. The quinoa adds complex carbs and fiber.

This recipe is gluten-free, and can be made dairy-free by omitting the mozzarella cheese. The combination of protein, fiber, and low-glycemic ingredients can help support hormone balance and reproductive health.

60. Lentil Tacos with Avocado

Ingredients:
- 1 cup dry brown or green lentils, rinsed
- 2 cups vegetable or chicken broth
- 1 tsp ground cumin
- 1 tsp chili powder
- 1/2 tsp garlic powder
- Salt and black pepper to taste
- 8-10 small corn tortillas or lettuce wraps
- 1 avocado, diced
- 1/4 cup diced red onion
- 2 tbsp chopped fresh cilantro
- Lime wedges for serving

Instructions:

1. In a medium saucepan, combine the rinsed lentils and broth. Bring to a boil over high heat.

2. Once boiling, reduce the heat to low, cover, and simmer for 15-20 minutes, or until the lentils are tender and the liquid is absorbed.

3. Remove the lentils from heat and stir in the cumin, chili powder, garlic powder, salt, and black pepper.

4. Warm the corn tortillas or prepare the lettuce wraps according to package instructions.

5. Spoon the seasoned lentils into the tortillas or lettuce wraps.

6. Top each taco with diced avocado, red onion, and chopped cilantro.

7. Serve the lentil tacos with lime wedges for squeezing over the top.

These lentil tacos with avocado are a delicious and nutritious option for a PCOS fertility diet. Lentils are a great source of plant-based protein, fiber, and complex carbs. The avocado provides healthy fats, and the minimal use of oil keeps the dish light.

This recipe is gluten-free, dairy-free, and vegan, making it suitable for various dietary needs. The combination of protein, fiber, and low-glycemic ingredients can help support hormone balance and reproductive health.

61. Berry Smoothie Bowl with Granola

Ingredients:
- 1 cup frozen mixed berries (such as strawberries, blueberries, raspberries)
- 1 cup unsweetened almond milk
- 1/2 cup plain Greek yogurt
- 1 tbsp chia seeds
- 1 tsp honey or maple syrup (optional)
- 1/4 cup homemade or store-bought granola
- Fresh berries for topping (optional)

Instructions:

1. In a high-speed blender, combine the frozen mixed berries, almond milk, Greek yogurt, and chia seeds. Blend until smooth and creamy.

2. Taste the smoothie and add the honey or maple syrup if desired, blending again briefly to incorporate.

3. Pour the berry smoothie into a bowl.

4. Sprinkle the granola over the top of the smoothie.

5. Garnish with additional fresh berries, if desired. Serve the berry smoothie bowl immediately.

This berry smoothie bowl is a nutritious and satisfying breakfast or snack option for a PCOS fertility diet. The frozen berries provide antioxidants, fiber, and natural sweetness, while the Greek yogurt offers protein and probiotics.

The chia seeds add healthy omega-3 fatty acids, and the granola provides a crunchy texture and additional fiber and nutrients. The minimal use of sweetener (honey or maple syrup) keeps the dish low in added sugars.

This recipe is gluten-free, and can be made dairy-free by using a non-dairy yogurt alternative. The combination of protein, fiber, and low-glycemic ingredients can help support hormone balance and reproductive health.

Enjoy this refreshing and nourishing berry smoothie bowl!

62. Savory Oatmeal with Spinach and Eggs

Ingredients:
- 1 cup rolled oats
- 2 cups unsweetened almond milk or low-sodium vegetable broth
- 2 cups fresh spinach, chopped
- 2 eggs
- 1 tbsp olive oil
- 1 clove garlic, minced
- 1/4 tsp ground cumin
- Salt and black pepper to taste
- Chopped fresh parsley for garnish (optional)

Instructions:
1. In a medium saucepan, bring the almond milk or vegetable broth to a boil over high heat. Stir in the rolled oats, reduce heat to low, and simmer for 5-7 minutes, stirring occasionally, until the oats are tender and the liquid is absorbed.

2. Remove the oatmeal from heat and stir in the chopped spinach until it's wilted.

3. In a small skillet, heat the olive oil over medium heat. Crack the eggs into the skillet and cook until the whites are set but the yolks are still runny, about 2-3 minutes.

4. Divide the savory oatmeal and spinach mixture between two bowls. Top each serving with a fried egg.

5. Sprinkle the oatmeal with the minced garlic, ground cumin, salt, and black pepper.

6. Garnish with chopped fresh parsley, if desired.

This savory oatmeal with spinach and eggs is a nutritious and satisfying breakfast option for a PCOS fertility diet. The oats provide complex carbs and fiber, while the eggs offer protein. The spinach adds vitamins, minerals, and antioxidants.

The recipe is gluten-free, dairy-free, and can be made vegan by omitting the eggs. The combination of protein, fiber, and low-glycemic ingredients can help support hormone balance and reproductive health.

Enjoy this savory and nourishing oatmeal dish as a delicious way to start your day!

63. Pumpkin Spice Overnight Oats

Ingredients:
- 1 cup rolled oats
- 1 cup unsweetened almond milk
- 1/2 cup canned pumpkin puree
- 2 tbsp chia seeds
- 1 tbsp maple syrup (optional)
- 1 tsp ground cinnamon
- 1/2 tsp ground ginger
- 1/4 tsp ground nutmeg
- 1/4 tsp ground cloves
- Pinch of salt

Instructions:

1. In a medium bowl, combine the rolled oats, almond milk, pumpkin puree, chia seeds, maple syrup (if using), cinnamon, ginger, nutmeg, cloves, and salt. Stir until well mixed.

2. Cover the bowl and refrigerate for at least 4 hours, or overnight.

3. When ready to serve, give the overnight oats a stir. You can enjoy them chilled or gently warmed.

4. Top the pumpkin spice overnight oats with additional almond milk, chopped nuts, or a drizzle of maple syrup, if desired.

These pumpkin spice overnight oats are a delicious and nutritious breakfast option for a PCOS fertility diet. The rolled oats provide complex carbs and fiber, while the pumpkin puree adds natural sweetness, vitamins, and antioxidants.

The chia seeds offer healthy omega-3 fatty acids, and the warming spices like cinnamon, ginger, and nutmeg can help support digestion.

This recipe is gluten-free, dairy-free, and can be made vegan by using maple syrup instead of honey. The combination of fiber, protein, and low-glycemic ingredients can help support hormone balance and reproductive health.

Enjoy these cozy and nourishing pumpkin spice overnight oats!

64. Whole Wheat Bagel with Lox and Avocado

Ingredients:
- 1 whole wheat bagel, toasted
- 2 oz smoked salmon (lox)
- 1/2 avocado, sliced
- 1 tbsp cream cheese (optional)
- 1 tbsp capers (optional)
- Freshly ground black pepper
- Lemon wedges for serving

Instructions:
1. Toast the whole wheat bagel until lightly golden.

2. Spread the toasted bagel with cream cheese, if using.

3. Layer the smoked salmon (lox) over the cream cheese.

4. Top the salmon with sliced avocado.

5. Sprinkle the capers over the avocado, if using.

6. Finish with a generous amount of freshly ground black pepper.

7. Serve the whole wheat bagel with lox and avocado with lemon wedges on the side.

This whole wheat bagel with lox and avocado is a nutritious and satisfying breakfast or brunch option for a PCOS fertility diet. The whole wheat bagel provides complex carbs and fiber, while the smoked salmon offers heart-healthy omega-3 fatty acids and protein.

The avocado adds healthy monounsaturated fats, fiber, and vitamins. The optional cream cheese and capers provide additional flavor and nutrients.

This recipe is gluten-free (if using a gluten-free bagel) and can be made dairy-free by omitting the cream cheese. The combination of protein, healthy fats, and low-glycemic ingredients can help support hormone balance and reproductive health.

Enjoy this delicious and nourishing whole wheat bagel with lox and avocado!

65. Egg Muffins with Vegetables

Ingredients:
- 8 eggs
- 1/2 cup unsweetened almond milk
- 1 cup diced bell peppers
- 1 cup diced spinach or kale
- 1/4 cup diced onion
- 2 tbsp grated Parmesan cheese (optional)
- Salt and black pepper to taste

Instructions:

1. Preheat the oven to 375°F. Grease a 12-cup muffin tin or line it with silicone or paper liners.

2. In a large bowl, whisk the eggs and almond milk together until well combined.

3. Stir in the diced bell peppers, spinach/kale, and onion. Season with salt and black pepper.

4. Divide the egg mixture evenly among the prepared muffin cups, filling each about 3/4 full.

5. If using, sprinkle the grated Parmesan cheese over the top of the egg muffins.

6. Bake for 20-25 minutes, or until the egg muffins are set and lightly golden on top.

7. Allow the egg muffins to cool in the tin for 5 minutes before removing them.

8. Serve the egg muffins warm or at room temperature.

These egg muffins with vegetables are a great make-ahead breakfast or snack option for a PCOS fertility diet. The eggs provide protein, while the vegetables offer fiber, vitamins, and minerals.

The recipe is gluten-free, and can be made dairy-free by omitting the Parmesan cheese. The combination of protein, fiber, and low-glycemic ingredients can help support hormone balance and reproductive health.

Enjoy these portable and nutritious egg muffins as a convenient and satisfying option throughout the week.

66. Mango Chia Pudding

Ingredients:
- 1 cup unsweetened almond milk
- 1/4 cup chia seeds
- 1 cup diced fresh mango
- 1 tbsp honey or maple syrup (optional)
- 1/2 tsp vanilla extract
- 1/4 tsp ground cinnamon

Instructions:

1. In a medium bowl, whisk together the almond milk and chia seeds. Cover and refrigerate for at least 2 hours, or overnight, stirring occasionally, until the mixture has thickened into a pudding-like consistency.

2. Once the chia pudding has set, stir in the diced mango, honey/maple syrup (if using), vanilla extract, and ground cinnamon.

3. Divide the mango chia pudding into individual serving bowls or jars.

4. Refrigerate the pudding until ready to serve, or enjoy it immediately.

This mango chia pudding is a delicious and nutritious snack or breakfast option for a PCOS fertility diet. The chia seeds provide fiber, protein, and omega-3 fatty acids, while the mango adds natural sweetness, vitamins, and antioxidants.

The recipe is gluten-free, dairy-free, and can be made vegan by using maple syrup instead of honey. The minimal added sweetener keeps the dish low in added sugars.

The combination of fiber, healthy fats, and low-glycemic ingredients in this mango chia pudding can help support hormone balance and reproductive health. Enjoy this refreshing and nourishing treat!

67. Protein-Packed Smoothie with Greek Yogurt

Ingredients:
- 1 cup unsweetened almond milk
- 1/2 cup plain Greek yogurt
- 1 scoop vanilla or unflavored protein powder
- 1 cup frozen mixed berries
- 1 tbsp almond butter
- 1 tbsp chia seeds
- 1 tsp honey or maple syrup (optional)

Instructions:
1. In a high-speed blender, combine the almond milk, Greek yogurt, protein powder, frozen mixed berries, almond butter, and chia seeds.

2. Blend on high speed until the mixture is smooth and creamy.

3. Taste the smoothie and add the honey or maple syrup, if desired, blending again briefly to incorporate.

4. Pour the protein-packed smoothie into a glass and enjoy immediately.

This smoothie is a nutritious and satisfying option for a PCOS fertility diet. The Greek yogurt provides protein and probiotics, while the almond milk, berries, and nut butter offer healthy fats, fiber, and antioxidants.

The addition of protein powder helps to make this smoothie more filling and supportive of muscle health. The chia seeds contribute omega-3 fatty acids, fiber, and additional protein.

This recipe is gluten-free, and can be made dairy-free by using a non-dairy yogurt alternative. The combination of protein, healthy fats, and low-glycemic ingredients can help support hormone balance and reproductive health.

Enjoy this protein-packed smoothie as a nutritious breakfast or snack!

68. Banana Nut Oatmeal

Ingredients:
- 1 cup rolled oats
- 1 1/2 cups unsweetened almond milk
- 1 ripe banana, mashed
- 2 tbsp chopped walnuts
- 1 tbsp chia seeds
- 1 tsp ground cinnamon
- 1/4 tsp ground nutmeg
- 1 tbsp almond butter (optional)
- Sliced banana for topping (optional)

Instructions:

1. In a medium saucepan, combine the rolled oats and almond milk. Bring to a simmer over medium heat, stirring occasionally.

2. Once the oats have softened and the mixture has thickened, about 5-7 minutes, remove from heat.

3. Stir in the mashed banana, chopped walnuts, chia seeds, cinnamon, and nutmeg until well combined.

4. If using, stir in the almond butter until it's melted and incorporated.

5. Serve the banana nut oatmeal warm, topped with sliced banana, if desired.

This banana nut oatmeal is a delicious and nutritious breakfast option for a PCOS fertility diet. The rolled oats provide complex carbs and fiber, while the banana adds natural sweetness, potassium, and antioxidants.

The walnuts offer healthy fats and protein, and the chia seeds contribute fiber, protein, and omega-3 fatty acids. The cinnamon and nutmeg provide additional flavor and health benefits.

This recipe is gluten-free, dairy-free, and can be made vegan by omitting the optional almond butter. The combination of fiber, protein, and low-glycemic ingredients can help support hormone balance and reproductive health.

Enjoy this comforting and nourishing banana nut oatmeal to start your day!

69. Cottage Cheese Pancakes

Ingredients:
- 1 cup low-fat cottage cheese
- 3 eggs
- 1/4 cup almond flour
- 1 tsp baking powder
- 1/4 tsp ground cinnamon
- 1 tbsp honey or maple syrup (optional)
- Coconut oil or avocado oil for cooking
- Fresh berries for serving (optional)

Instructions:
1. In a medium bowl, combine the cottage cheese, eggs, almond flour, baking powder, and cinnamon. Whisk until the mixture is well blended and smooth.

2. If using, stir in the honey or maple syrup.

3. Heat a large non-stick skillet or griddle over medium heat and lightly grease with coconut oil or avocado oil.

4. Scoop the cottage cheese batter onto the hot skillet, forming pancakes about 3-4 inches in diameter.

5. Cook the pancakes for 2-3 minutes per side, or until they are golden brown and cooked through.

6. Serve the cottage cheese pancakes warm, topped with fresh berries if desired.

These cottage cheese pancakes are a protein-packed and nutrient-dense option for a PCOS fertility diet. The cottage cheese provides a good source of protein, while the almond flour and eggs help to create a fluffy texture.

The recipe is gluten-free and can be made dairy-free by using a non-dairy cottage cheese alternative. The minimal use of sweetener (honey or maple syrup) keeps the dish low in added sugars.

The combination of protein, fiber, and low-glycemic ingredients in these cottage cheese pancakes can help support hormone balance and reproductive health. Enjoy this satisfying and nourishing breakfast!

70. Spinach and Cheese Frittata

Ingredients:
- 8 eggs
- 1/4 cup unsweetened almond milk
- 1/2 tsp dried oregano
- 1/4 tsp garlic powder
- Salt and black pepper to taste
- 2 cups fresh spinach, chopped
- 1/2 cup shredded mozzarella or feta cheese
- 1 tbsp olive oil

Instructions:
1. Preheat the oven to 375°F.

2. In a medium bowl, whisk together the eggs, almond milk, oregano, garlic powder, salt, and black pepper.

3. Heat the olive oil in a 9-inch oven-safe skillet over medium heat.

4. Add the chopped spinach to the skillet and sauté for 2-3 minutes, until wilted.

5. Pour the egg mixture over the spinach and sprinkle the shredded cheese on top.

6. Transfer the skillet to the preheated oven and bake for 18-22 minutes, or until the frittata is set and the cheese is melted.

7. Remove the frittata from the oven and let it cool for 5 minutes before slicing and serving.

This spinach and cheese frittata is a delicious and nutritious option for a PCOS fertility diet. The eggs provide protein, while the spinach offers fiber, vitamins, and minerals. The cheese adds a creamy texture and a boost of calcium.

The recipe is gluten-free and can be made dairy-free by using a non-dairy cheese alternative. The combination of protein, fiber, and low-glycemic ingredients can help support hormone balance and reproductive health.

Enjoy this savory and satisfying spinach and cheese frittata for breakfast, brunch, or even a light dinner.

71. Trail Mix with Dried Fruits and Nuts

Ingredients:
- 1 cup raw almonds
- 1 cup raw walnuts
- 1/2 cup raw pumpkin seeds
- 1/2 cup raw sunflower seeds
- 1/2 cup unsweetened dried cranberries
- 1/2 cup unsweetened dried apricots, chopped
- 1/4 cup unsweetened shredded coconut

Instructions:
1. In a large bowl, combine the almonds, walnuts, pumpkin seeds, sunflower seeds, dried cranberries, dried apricots, and shredded coconut.

2. Stir to mix well.

3. Store the trail mix in an airtight container at room temperature for up to 2 weeks.

This trail mix is a great source of healthy fats, fiber, and antioxidants, which can be beneficial for women with PCOS who are trying to conceive. The nuts and seeds provide protein, healthy fats, and minerals like magnesium and zinc, while the dried fruits add natural sweetness and additional nutrients.

Remember, it's always a good idea to consult with a healthcare professional, such as a registered dietitian or your doctor, to develop a personalized PCOS fertility diet plan that takes into account your specific needs and health conditions.

72. Roasted Chickpeas

Ingredients:
- 1 (15 oz) can of chickpeas (garbanzo beans), drained and rinsed
- 1 tbsp olive oil
- 1 tsp ground cumin
- 1/2 tsp paprika
- 1/4 tsp garlic powder
- 1/4 tsp salt
- 1/4 tsp black pepper

Instructions:
1. Preheat your oven to 400°F (200°C).

2. Pat the drained and rinsed chickpeas dry with a paper towel or clean kitchen towel.

3. In a medium bowl, toss the chickpeas with the olive oil, cumin, paprika, garlic powder, salt, and black pepper until they are evenly coated.

4. Spread the seasoned chickpeas in a single layer on a baking sheet lined with parchment paper.

5. Roast the chickpeas in the preheated oven for 20-25 minutes, stirring halfway, until they are crispy and golden brown.

6. Allow the roasted chickpeas to cool for a few minutes before serving.

Chickpeas are a great source of protein, fiber, and complex carbohydrates, which can be beneficial for women with PCOS who are trying to conceive. The roasting process also helps to enhance the nutty flavor and crispy texture of the chickpeas.

You can enjoy the roasted chickpeas as a snack or add them to salads, bowls, or other dishes. Remember to consult with a healthcare professional to develop a personalized PCOS fertility diet plan that meets your specific needs.

73. Almonds and Dark Chocolate

ingredients:
- 1 cup raw, unsalted almonds
- 1 oz dark chocolate (70% cacao or higher), chopped

Instructions:
1. In a small bowl, combine the raw almonds and chopped dark chocolate.

2. Mix the ingredients together until the chocolate is evenly distributed among the almonds.

3. Enjoy the almonds and dark chocolate as a snack.

This combination of almonds and dark chocolate provides a variety of nutrients that can be beneficial for women with PCOS who are trying to conceive:

Almonds:
- High in healthy fats, protein, fiber, and antioxidants
- May help improve insulin sensitivity and reduce inflammation

Dark Chocolate:
- Rich in antioxidants, such as flavonoids, that can help reduce inflammation
- May help improve insulin sensitivity and reduce the risk of gestational diabetes

The combination of the healthy fats, protein, and fiber from the almonds, along with the antioxidants and potential insulin-sensitizing effects of the dark chocolate, make this a great snack option for a PCOS fertility diet.

Remember to choose dark chocolate with a high cacao content (70% or higher) and to consume this snack in moderation as part of a balanced diet. As always, it's best to consult with a healthcare professional to develop a personalized PCOS fertility diet plan.

74. Bell Pepper Slices with Guacamole

Ingredients:
For the Guacamole:
- 2 ripe avocados, pitted and mashed
- 1 tablespoon fresh lime juice
- 1 clove garlic, minced
- 2 tablespoons diced red onion
- 2 tablespoons chopped cilantro (optional)
- 1/4 teaspoon salt
- 1/4 teaspoon ground cumin

For the Bell Pepper Slices:
- 1 red bell pepper, sliced into thin strips
- 1 yellow bell pepper, sliced into thin strips

Instructions:
1. In a medium bowl, mash the avocados with a fork or potato masher.

2. Add the lime juice, garlic, red onion, cilantro (if using), salt, and cumin. Stir to combine.

3. Arrange the bell pepper slices on a serving platter or plate.

4. Scoop the guacamole onto the bell pepper slices and serve.

This snack is a great option for a PCOS fertility diet for several reasons:

1. Bell peppers are a good source of vitamins, minerals, and antioxidants, which can help support overall health and fertility.

2. Avocados are rich in healthy monounsaturated fats, fiber, and various vitamins and minerals that are important for fertility, such as folate, vitamin E, and zinc.

3. The combination of the crunchy bell peppers and the creamy, flavorful guacamole provides a satisfying and nutrient-dense snack.

Remember to consult with a healthcare professional, such as a registered dietitian or your doctor, to develop a personalized PCOS fertility diet plan that takes into account your specific needs and health conditions.

75. Fruit Skewers

Ingredients:
- 1 cup cubed watermelon
- 1 cup cubed pineapple
- 1 cup cubed mango
- 1 cup cubed kiwi
- 1 cup halved strawberries
- Wooden skewers

Instructions:
1. Wash and prepare the fruit. Cut the watermelon, pineapple, mango, and kiwi into 1-inch cubes. Halve the strawberries.

2. Thread the fruit onto the wooden skewers, alternating the different types of fruit.

3. Arrange the fruit skewers on a serving platter or plate.

4. Serve chilled or at room temperature.

These fruit skewers are a great option for a PCOS fertility diet for several reasons:

1. Variety of fruits: The combination of watermelon, pineapple, mango, kiwi, and strawberries provides a wide range of vitamins, minerals, and antioxidants that are important for overall health and fertility.

2. Low glycemic index: Many of the fruits used, such as berries, kiwi, and watermelon, have a relatively low glycemic index, which can help manage blood sugar levels and support fertility.

3. Hydration: Fruits like watermelon and pineapple are high in water content, which can help with hydration and overall health.

4. Convenience: The skewers make for a portable and easy-to-eat snack or side dish.

Remember to consult with a healthcare professional, such as a registered dietitian or your doctor, to develop a personalized PCOS fertility diet plan that takes into account your specific needs and health conditions.

76. Mini Caprese Salad Bites

Ingredients:
- 12 cherry tomatoes, halved
- 12 small fresh mozzarella balls (or use mozzarella pearls)
- 12 fresh basil leaves
- 2 tablespoons balsamic glaze
- Salt and pepper to taste

Instructions:
1. Arrange the cherry tomato halves on a serving platter or plate.

2. Top each tomato half with a small mozzarella ball.

3. Place a fresh basil leaf on top of each mozzarella ball.

4. Drizzle the balsamic glaze over the top of the mini caprese salad bites.

5. Season with a pinch of salt and pepper, if desired.

These mini caprese salad bites are a great option for a PCOS fertility diet for several reasons:

1. Tomatoes: Tomatoes are a good source of lycopene, an antioxidant that may help improve fertility and reproductive health.

2. Mozzarella: Mozzarella cheese is a source of protein and calcium, both of which are important for fertility and overall health.

3. Basil: Basil is a herb that contains antioxidants and anti-inflammatory properties, which can be beneficial for women with PCOS.

4. Balsamic glaze: Balsamic vinegar has been shown to have potential benefits for insulin sensitivity and PCOS management.

5. Portion control: The mini size of these bites makes it easy to enjoy a satisfying and nutrient-dense snack or appetizer without overindulging.

Remember to consult with a healthcare professional, such as a registered dietitian or your doctor, to develop a personalized PCOS fertility diet plan that takes into account your specific needs and health conditions.

77. Avocado Deviled Eggs

Ingredients:
- 6 hard-boiled eggs, peeled
- 1 ripe avocado, pitted and mashed
- 1 tablespoon Dijon mustard
- 1 tablespoon fresh lemon juice
- 1/4 teaspoon salt
- 1/8 teaspoon black pepper
- Paprika for garnish (optional)

Instructions:
1. Cut the hard-boiled eggs in half lengthwise and carefully remove the yolks, placing them in a medium bowl.

2. In the bowl with the egg yolks, mash the avocado until smooth and well combined.

3. Add the Dijon mustard, lemon juice, salt, and black pepper. Mix well until the filling is creamy and well-seasoned.

4. Spoon or pipe the avocado filling back into the egg white halves. Sprinkle the deviled eggs with a light dusting of paprika, if desired. Chill the deviled eggs in the refrigerator for at least 30 minutes before serving.

These avocado deviled eggs are a great option for a PCOS fertility diet for several reasons:

1. Eggs: Eggs are a excellent source of protein, vitamins, and minerals that are important for fertility and overall health.

2. Avocado: Avocados are rich in healthy monounsaturated fats, fiber, and various vitamins and minerals that can support fertility, such as folate, vitamin E, and zinc.

3. Dijon mustard and lemon juice: These ingredients add flavor and may also have anti-inflammatory properties that can be beneficial for women with PCOS.

4. Portion control: The deviled egg format provides a satisfying and nutrient-dense snack or appetizer in a controlled portion size.

Remember to consult with a healthcare professional, such as a registered dietitian or your doctor, to develop a personalized PCOS fertility diet plan that takes into account your specific needs and health conditions.

78. Pumpkin Seeds

1. Nutrient-dense: Pumpkin seeds are a great source of various vitamins and minerals that are important for fertility and overall health, such as zinc, magnesium, iron, and B vitamins.

2. High in protein and healthy fats: Pumpkin seeds are a good source of plant-based protein and healthy unsaturated fats, which can help support hormone balance and fertility.

3. Anti-inflammatory properties: Pumpkin seeds contain antioxidants and anti-inflammatory compounds that may help reduce inflammation, which is often a concern for women with PCOS.

4. Potential benefits for PCOS: Some studies have suggested that pumpkin seed oil may help improve insulin sensitivity and reduce androgen levels in women with PCOS, which can be beneficial for fertility.

You can enjoy pumpkin seeds in a variety of ways, such as:

- Roasted pumpkin seeds as a snack

- Sprinkled on top of salads, yogurt, or oatmeal

- Incorporated into homemade trail mixes or energy bars

- Ground into a powder and used in baking or as a breading for proteins

When incorporating pumpkin seeds into your PCOS fertility diet, be mindful of portion sizes, as they are calorie-dense. Consult with a healthcare professional, such as a registered dietitian or your doctor, to develop a personalized diet plan that meets your specific needs and health conditions.

79. Greek Yogurt and Berry Parfait

Ingredients:
- 2 cups plain Greek yogurt
- 1 cup fresh or frozen mixed berries (such as blueberries, raspberries, and blackberries)
- 2 tablespoons chopped walnuts or almonds (optional)
- 1 tablespoon honey or maple syrup (optional)

Instructions:

1. In a parfait glass or small bowl, layer the Greek yogurt and mixed berries, starting and ending with the yogurt.

2. If using, sprinkle the chopped nuts over the top of the parfait.

3. Drizzle the honey or maple syrup over the top, if desired.
4. Serve chilled.

This Greek yogurt and berry parfait is an excellent choice for a PCOS fertility diet for several reasons:

1. Greek yogurt: Greek yogurt is a great source of protein, which can help support fertility and overall health. It also contains probiotics that may help improve gut health.

2. Berries: Berries are rich in antioxidants, fiber, and vitamins that are important for fertility, such as vitamin C and folate.

3. Nuts (optional): Walnuts and almonds provide healthy fats, protein, and additional nutrients like magnesium and zinc, which are beneficial for fertility.

4. Honey or maple syrup (optional): These natural sweeteners can provide a touch of sweetness without the blood sugar spike of refined sugars.

This parfait can be enjoyed as a healthy breakfast, snack, or dessert. Remember to consult with a healthcare professional, such as a registered dietitian or your doctor, to develop a personalized PCOS fertility diet plan that takes into account your specific needs and health conditions.

80. Edamame Hummus with Veggies

Ingredients:
For the Edamame Hummus:
- 1 cup shelled edamame, cooked and cooled
- 2 tablespoons tahini
- 2 tablespoons fresh lemon juice
- 1 clove garlic, minced
- 1/4 teaspoon ground cumin
- 1/4 teaspoon salt
- 2-3 tablespoons water, as needed to blend

For the Veggie Dippers:
- 1 cup sliced cucumber
- 1 cup sliced bell pepper
- 1 cup baby carrots

Instructions:
1. In a food processor or high-powered blender, combine the cooked edamame, tahini, lemon juice, garlic, cumin, and salt. Blend until smooth, adding 2-3 tablespoons of water as needed to reach your desired consistency.

2. Transfer the edamame hummus to a serving bowl.

3. Arrange the sliced cucumber, bell pepper, and baby carrots around the hummus, creating a veggie platter. Serve the edamame hummus with the fresh vegetables.

This edamame hummus with veggies is a great option for a PCOS fertility diet for several reasons:

1. Edamame: Edamame is a good source of plant-based protein, fiber, and various vitamins and minerals that are important for fertility, such as folate and iron.

2. Tahini: Tahini, a paste made from ground sesame seeds, provides healthy fats and minerals like calcium and magnesium.

3. Vegetables: The fresh vegetables, such as cucumber, bell pepper, and carrots, are low in carbohydrates and high in fiber, vitamins, and antioxidants that can support overall health and fertility.

4. Balanced macronutrients: The combination of protein, healthy fats, and fiber-rich carbohydrates can help manage blood sugar levels and support fertility.

81. Mediterranean Quinoa Bowl

Ingredients:

- 1 cup uncooked quinoa, rinsed
- 2 cups low-sodium vegetable
or chicken broth
- 1 cup cherry tomatoes, halved
- 1 cup cucumber, diced
- 1/2 cup crumbled feta cheese
- 1/4 cup kalamata olives, sliced

- 2 tablespoons chopped fresh parsley
- 2 tablespoons olive oil
- 2 tablespoons lemon juice
- 1 clove garlic, minced
- 1/4 teaspoon salt
- 1/4 teaspoon black pepper

Instructions:

1. In a medium saucepan, combine the quinoa and broth. Bring to a boil, then reduce heat to low, cover, and simmer for 15-20 minutes, or until the quinoa is cooked and the liquid is absorbed.

2. Transfer the cooked quinoa to a large bowl and let it cool slightly.

3. Add the cherry tomatoes, cucumber, feta cheese, olives, and parsley to the bowl with the quinoa.

4. In a small bowl, whisk together the olive oil, lemon juice, garlic, salt, and black pepper.

5. Pour the dressing over the quinoa and vegetable mixture and toss gently to combine. Serve the Mediterranean quinoa bowl warm or chilled.

This Mediterranean quinoa bowl is a great option for a PCOS fertility diet for several reasons:

1. Quinoa: Quinoa is a gluten-free, high-protein grain that is a good source of fiber, vitamins, and minerals, which are important for fertility.

2. Vegetables: The cherry tomatoes, cucumber, and olives provide a variety of vitamins, minerals, and antioxidants that can support overall health and fertility.

3. Feta cheese: Feta cheese is a good source of protein and calcium, both of which are important for fertility.

4. Healthy fats: The olive oil in the dressing provides healthy monounsaturated fats that can help support hormone balance and fertility.

82. Chicken and Avocado Salad

Ingredients:
- 2 cups cooked, shredded or diced chicken breast
- 1 ripe avocado, diced
- 1/2 cup diced celery
- 1/4 cup diced red onion
- 2 tablespoons chopped fresh cilantro (or parsley)
- 2 tablespoons olive oil
- 1 tablespoon lemon juice
- 1/4 teaspoon salt
- 1/4 teaspoon black pepper

Instructions:
1. In a large bowl, combine the cooked chicken, diced avocado, celery, red onion, and chopped cilantro (or parsley).

2. In a small bowl, whisk together the olive oil, lemon juice, salt, and black pepper.

3. Pour the dressing over the chicken and avocado mixture and gently toss to coat.

4. Serve the chicken and avocado salad on a bed of greens, in a lettuce wrap, or with whole-grain crackers or bread.

This chicken and avocado salad is a great option for a PCOS fertility diet for several reasons:

1. Chicken: Chicken is a lean protein source that can help support muscle development and overall health.

2. Avocado: Avocados are rich in healthy monounsaturated fats, fiber, and various vitamins and minerals that are important for fertility, such as folate, vitamin E, and zinc.

3. Vegetables: The celery and red onion provide additional nutrients and fiber, which can help support overall health and fertility.

4. Healthy fats and antioxidants: The olive oil and lemon juice in the dressing provide healthy fats and antioxidants that can help reduce inflammation and support fertility.

Remember to consult with a healthcare professional, such as a registered dietitian or your doctor, to develop a personalized PCOS fertility diet plan that takes into account your specific needs and health conditions.

83. Vegan Buddha Bowl

Ingredients:
- 1 cup cooked quinoa
- 1 cup roasted sweet potato cubes
- 1 cup roasted chickpeas
- 1 cup shredded kale or spinach
- 1/2 cup sliced avocado
- 2 tablespoons toasted pumpkin seeds
- 2 tablespoons tahini dressing (see below)

For the Tahini Dressing:
- 2 tablespoons tahini
- 1 tablespoon lemon juice
- 1 tablespoon water
- 1 teaspoon maple syrup
- 1/4 teaspoon ground cumin
- 1/4 teaspoon salt

Instructions:

1. Prepare the quinoa according to package instructions and set aside.

2. Roast the sweet potato cubes and chickpeas in the oven at 400°F for 20-25 minutes, or until tender and lightly browned.

3. In a large bowl, layer the cooked quinoa, roasted sweet potato, roasted chickpeas, shredded kale or spinach, and sliced avocado. Sprinkle the toasted pumpkin seeds over the top.

4. In a small bowl, whisk together all the ingredients for the tahini dressing. Drizzle the tahini dressing over the Buddha bowl and serve.

This vegan Buddha bowl is a great option for a PCOS fertility diet for several reasons:

1. Quinoa: Quinoa is a gluten-free, high-protein grain that is a good source of fiber, vitamins, and minerals, which are important for fertility.

2. Sweet potato and chickpeas: These provide complex carbohydrates, fiber, and a variety of vitamins and minerals that can support overall health and fertility.

3. Kale or spinach: These leafy greens are rich in antioxidants, folate, and other nutrients that are important for fertility.

4. Avocado and pumpkin seeds: These provide healthy fats, protein, and additional nutrients like zinc and magnesium, which are beneficial for fertility.

5. Tahini dressing: Tahini is a good source of healthy fats and minerals that can help support hormone balance and fertility.

84. Spinach and Strawberry Salad

Ingredients:
- 5 cups fresh spinach leaves, washed and dried
- 1 cup fresh strawberries, sliced
- 1/4 cup raw walnuts, chopped
- 2 tablespoons crumbled feta cheese
- 2 tablespoons balsamic vinegar
- 1 tablespoon extra-virgin olive oil
- 1 teaspoon Dijon mustard
- 1 teaspoon honey
- 1/4 teaspoon salt
- 1/8 teaspoon black pepper

Instructions:
1. In a large salad bowl, combine the spinach, sliced strawberries, chopped walnuts, and crumbled feta cheese.

2. In a small bowl, whisk together the balsamic vinegar, olive oil, Dijon mustard, honey, salt, and black pepper to make the dressing.

3. Drizzle the dressing over the salad and toss gently to coat. Serve the spinach and strawberry salad immediately.

This spinach and strawberry salad is a great option for a PCOS fertility diet for several reasons:

1. Spinach: Spinach is a nutrient-dense leafy green that is rich in folate, iron, and antioxidants, all of which are important for fertility.

2. Strawberries: Strawberries are a good source of vitamin C, fiber, and antioxidants that can help support overall health and fertility.

3. Walnuts: Walnuts are a great source of omega-3 fatty acids, which can help reduce inflammation and support fertility.

4. Feta cheese: Feta cheese is a good source of protein and calcium, both of which are important for fertility.

5. Balsamic vinegar and olive oil: The combination of balsamic vinegar and olive oil in the dressing provides healthy fats and antioxidants that can help support fertility.

85. Roasted Beet and Goat Cheese Salad

Ingredients:
- 3 medium beets, peeled and
  cut into 1-inch cubes
- 1 tablespoon olive oil
- 1/4 teaspoon salt
- 1/8 teaspoon black pepper
- 5 cups mixed greens (such as spinach, arugula, or kale)
- 2 ounces crumbled goat cheese
- 2 tablespoons toasted walnuts or pecans
- 2 tablespoons balsamic vinegar
- 1 tablespoon extra-virgin olive oil

Instructions:

1. Preheat your oven to 400°F (200°C).

2. Toss the cubed beets with 1 tablespoon of olive oil, salt, and black pepper. Spread the beets on a baking sheet and roast for 20-25 minutes, or until tender and lightly caramelized.
3. Allow the roasted beets to cool slightly.

4. In a large salad bowl, combine the mixed greens, roasted beets, crumbled goat cheese, and toasted nuts.

5. In a small bowl, whisk together the balsamic vinegar and 1 tablespoon of extra-virgin olive oil to make the dressing. Drizzle the dressing over the salad and toss gently to coat. Serve the roasted beet and goat cheese salad immediately.

This roasted beet and goat cheese salad is a great option for a PCOS fertility diet for several reasons:

1. Beets: Beets are a good source of folate, fiber, and antioxidants, which can support overall health and fertility.

2. Goat cheese: Goat cheese is a good source of protein and calcium, both of which are important for fertility.

3. Greens: The mixed greens, such as spinach and arugula, provide a variety of vitamins, minerals, and antioxidants that can support fertility.

4. Nuts: The toasted walnuts or pecans add healthy fats, protein, and additional nutrients like magnesium and zinc, which are beneficial for fertility.

5. Balsamic vinegar and olive oil: The dressing provides healthy fats and antioxidants that can help reduce inflammation and support fertility.

86. Tuna Salad with Olive Oil and Lemon

Ingredients:
- 2 (5 oz) cans of tuna, drained and flaked
- 2 tablespoons extra-virgin olive oil
- 2 tablespoons fresh lemon juice
- 1/4 cup diced celery
- 2 tablespoons diced red onion
- 2 tablespoons chopped fresh parsley
- 1/4 teaspoon salt
- 1/8 teaspoon black pepper

Instructions:
1. In a medium bowl, combine the flaked tuna, olive oil, and lemon juice. Mix well to coat the tuna.

2. Add the diced celery, red onion, chopped parsley, salt, and black pepper. Stir to combine.

3. Serve the tuna salad on a bed of greens, in a lettuce wrap, or with whole-grain crackers or bread.

This tuna salad with olive oil and lemon is a great option for a PCOS fertility diet for several reasons:
1. Tuna: Tuna is a good source of lean protein, which can help support muscle development and overall health. It also contains omega-3 fatty acids, which can help reduce inflammation and support fertility.

2. Olive oil: The extra-virgin olive oil provides healthy monounsaturated fats that can help support hormone balance and fertility.

3. Lemon: Lemon juice is a good source of vitamin C, which can help support the immune system and overall health.

4. Vegetables: The celery and red onion provide additional nutrients and fiber, which can help support overall health and fertility.

5. Parsley: Parsley is a herb that contains antioxidants and anti-inflammatory properties, which can be beneficial for women with PCOS.

Remember to choose a low-mercury tuna variety and to consult with a healthcare professional, such as a registered dietitian or your doctor, to develop a personalized PCOS fertility diet plan that takes into account your specific needs and health conditions.

87. Brown Rice Sushi Rolls

Ingredients:
- 1 cup uncooked brown rice
- 2 cups water
- 1/4 cup rice vinegar
- 1 tablespoon honey
- 1/2 teaspoon salt
- 4 sheets of nori (seaweed sheets)
- 1 avocado, sliced
- 1 cucumber, peeled and cut into thin strips
- 1 carrot, peeled and cut into thin strips

Instructions:

1. Cook the brown rice: In a medium saucepan, combine the brown rice and water. Bring to a boil, then reduce heat to low, cover, and simmer for 25-30 minutes, or until the rice is tender and the water is absorbed.

2. Make the sushi rice: In a small bowl, combine the rice vinegar, honey, and salt. Pour this mixture over the cooked brown rice and stir gently to combine.

3. Lay a sheet of nori on a bamboo sushi mat or a clean, flat surface. Spread about 1/2 cup of the brown rice mixture evenly over the nori, leaving a 1-inch border at the top.

4. Arrange the avocado, cucumber, and carrot strips in a line across the center of the rice.

5. Carefully roll the sushi, using the bamboo mat or your hands to tightly roll the nori around the fillings.

6. Slice the rolled sushi into 6-8 pieces using a sharp, wet knife. Repeat the process with the remaining nori sheets and fillings. Serve the brown rice sushi rolls immediately.

These brown rice sushi rolls are a great option for a PCOS fertility diet for several reasons:

1. Brown rice: Brown rice is a whole grain that is a good source of fiber, vitamins, and minerals, which are important for fertility.

2. Avocado, cucumber, and carrot: These vegetables provide a variety of vitamins, minerals, and antioxidants that can support overall health and fertility.

3. Nori: Nori is a type of seaweed that is a good source of iodine, which is important for thyroid health and fertility.

4. Portion control: The sushi roll format allows for a satisfying and nutrient-dense meal or snack in a controlled portion size.

88. Cucumber and Tomato Salad with Feta

Ingredients:
- 2 cups diced cucumber
- 1 cup halved cherry tomatoes
- 1/4 cup crumbled feta cheese
- 2 tablespoons chopped fresh basil
- 1 tablespoon olive oil
- 1 tablespoon red wine vinegar
- 1/4 teaspoon salt
- 1/8 teaspoon black pepper

Instructions:
1. In a large bowl, combine the diced cucumber, halved cherry tomatoes, crumbled feta cheese, and chopped fresh basil.

2. In a small bowl, whisk together the olive oil, red wine vinegar, salt, and black pepper to make the dressing.

3. Pour the dressing over the cucumber and tomato mixture and toss gently to coat.

4. Serve the cucumber and tomato salad with feta immediately or chill in the refrigerator for 30 minutes before serving.

This cucumber and tomato salad with feta is a great option for a PCOS fertility diet for several reasons:

1. Cucumbers: Cucumbers are a good source of hydration, fiber, and various vitamins and minerals that can support overall health and fertility.

2. Tomatoes: Tomatoes are a rich source of lycopene, an antioxidant that may help improve fertility and reproductive health.

3. Feta cheese: Feta cheese is a good source of protein and calcium, both of which are important for fertility.

4. Basil: Basil is a herb that contains antioxidants and anti-inflammatory properties, which can be beneficial for women with PCOS.

5. Olive oil and vinegar: The dressing provides healthy fats and antioxidants that can help reduce inflammation and support fertility.

89. Grilled Chicken and Veggie Wrap

Ingredients:
- 4 oz grilled chicken breast, sliced or diced
- 1/2 cup sliced bell peppers
- 1/2 cup sliced cucumber
- 1/4 cup shredded spinach or kale
- 2 tablespoons hummus
- 1 whole-wheat tortilla or wrap

Instructions:

1. Grill or bake the chicken breast until cooked through and lightly charred. Allow to cool slightly, then slice or dice the chicken.

2. In the center of the tortilla or wrap, layer the grilled chicken, sliced bell peppers, sliced cucumber, and shredded spinach or kale.

3. Spread the hummus over the top of the vegetables.

4. Fold the bottom of the tortilla or wrap up over the filling, then fold in the sides and continue rolling tightly to create a wrap.

5. Slice the wrap in half diagonally and serve.

This grilled chicken and veggie wrap is a great option for a PCOS fertility diet for several reasons:

1. Grilled chicken: Chicken is a lean protein source that can help support muscle development and overall health. Grilling it adds a nice flavor without added oils or fats.

2. Vegetables: The bell peppers, cucumber, and spinach or kale provide a variety of vitamins, minerals, and antioxidants that can support fertility and overall health.

3. Hummus: Hummus is a good source of plant-based protein, fiber, and healthy fats that can help manage blood sugar levels and support fertility.

4. Whole-wheat tortilla: Using a whole-wheat tortilla or wrap provides complex carbohydrates, fiber, and additional nutrients that are important for fertility.

Remember to consult with a healthcare professional, such as a registered dietitian or your doctor, to develop a personalized PCOS fertility diet plan that takes into account your specific needs and health conditions.

90. Sweet Potato and Black Bean Salad

Ingredients:
- 2 tablespoons olive oil
- 2 tablespoons lime juice
- 1 teaspoon ground cumin
- 1/4 teaspoon salt
- 1/4 teaspoon black pepper

- 2 medium sweet potatoes, peeled and cubed
- 1 (15 oz) can black beans, rinsed and drained
- 1 cup diced red bell pepper
- 1/2 cup diced red onion
- 2 tablespoons chopped fresh cilantro

Instructions:
1. Preheat your oven to 400°F (200°C).

2. Toss the cubed sweet potatoes with 1 tablespoon of olive oil and spread them on a baking sheet. Roast for 20-25 minutes, or until the sweet potatoes are tender and lightly browned.

3. In a large bowl, combine the roasted sweet potatoes, black beans, diced red bell pepper, diced red onion, and chopped cilantro.

4. In a small bowl, whisk together the remaining 1 tablespoon of olive oil, lime juice, cumin, salt, and black pepper to make the dressing.

5. Pour the dressing over the sweet potato and black bean mixture and toss gently to coat.

6. Serve the sweet potato and black bean salad at room temperature or chilled.

This sweet potato and black bean salad is a great option for a PCOS fertility diet for several reasons:

1. Sweet potatoes: Sweet potatoes are a good source of complex carbohydrates, fiber, and various vitamins and minerals, including beta-carotene, which can support fertility.

2. Black beans: Black beans are a good source of plant-based protein, fiber, and folate, all of which are important for fertility.

3. Vegetables: The red bell pepper and red onion provide additional vitamins, minerals, and antioxidants that can support overall health and fertility.

4. Healthy fats: The olive oil in the dressing provides healthy monounsaturated fats that can help support hormone balance and fertility.

5. Spices: The cumin and lime juice in the dressing add flavor and may also have anti-inflammatory properties that can be beneficial for women with PCOS.

91. Grilled Lamb Chops with Mint

Ingredients:
- 4 lamb chops (about 1 lb total)
- 2 tablespoons olive oil
- 2 tablespoons fresh lemon juice
- 2 cloves garlic, minced
- 1 teaspoon dried oregano
- 1/4 teaspoon salt
- 1/4 teaspoon black pepper
- 2 tablespoons chopped fresh mint

Instructions:

1. In a shallow dish, combine the olive oil, lemon juice, garlic, oregano, salt, and black pepper. Add the lamb chops and turn to coat both sides with the marinade. Cover and refrigerate for 30 minutes to 1 hour.

2. Preheat your grill or grill pan to medium-high heat.

3. Remove the lamb chops from the marinade and grill for 3-4 minutes per side, or until they reach your desired level of doneness.

4. Transfer the grilled lamb chops to a serving plate and sprinkle with the chopped fresh mint. Serve the grilled lamb chops with mint immediately.

This grilled lamb chops with mint recipe is a great option for a PCOS fertility diet for several reasons:

1. Lamb: Lamb is a good source of protein, iron, and zinc, all of which are important for fertility and overall health.

2. Mint: Fresh mint contains antioxidants and anti-inflammatory properties that can be beneficial for women with PCOS.

3. Olive oil and lemon juice: The marinade provides healthy fats and vitamin C, which can help support fertility.

4. Garlic and oregano: These ingredients add flavor and may also have anti-inflammatory effects that can be helpful for PCOS.

Remember to choose lean cuts of lamb and to consult with a healthcare professional, such as a registered dietitian or your doctor, to develop a personalized PCOS fertility diet plan that takes into account your specific needs and health conditions.

92. Vegetable Lasagna with Zucchini Noodles

Ingredients:
- 1 teaspoon dried oregano
- 1/2 teaspoon dried basil
- 1/4 teaspoon red pepper flakes (optional)
- 1/2 teaspoon salt
- 1/4 teaspoon black pepper
- 1 cup part-skim ricotta cheese
- 1 cup shredded mozzarella cheese
- 3 medium zucchini, sliced lengthwise into thin noodle-like strips
- 1 tablespoon olive oil
- 1 onion, diced
- 3 cloves garlic, minced
- 1 red bell pepper, diced
- 8 oz sliced mushrooms
- 1 (28 oz) can crushed tomatoes
- 2 tablespoons tomato paste

Instructions:
1. Preheat your oven to 375°F (190°C).

2. In a large skillet, heat the olive oil over medium heat. Add the onion and garlic and sauté for 2-3 minutes until fragrant.

3. Add the diced bell pepper and sliced mushrooms to the skillet. Cook for 5-7 minutes, stirring occasionally, until the vegetables are tender.

4. Stir in the crushed tomatoes, tomato paste, oregano, basil, red pepper flakes (if using), salt, and black pepper. Simmer for 10 minutes, stirring occasionally.

5. In a 9x13 inch baking dish, layer half of the zucchini noodles, half of the vegetable tomato sauce, and half of the ricotta and mozzarella cheeses. Repeat the layers.

6. Cover the baking dish with foil and bake for 30 minutes. Remove the foil and bake for an additional 10-15 minutes, or until the cheese is melted and bubbly. Let the lasagna cool for 5-10 minutes before serving.

This vegetable lasagna with zucchini noodles is a great option for a PCOS fertility diet for several reasons:

1. Zucchini noodles: Using zucchini noodles instead of traditional pasta provides a low-carb, high-fiber alternative that can help manage blood sugar levels.

2. Vegetables: The onion, bell pepper, mushrooms, and tomatoes provide a variety of vitamins, minerals, and antioxidants that can support fertility and overall health.

3. Ricotta and mozzarella: These cheeses are good sources of protein and calcium, which are important for fertility.

93. Chicken and Veggie Stir-Fry

Ingredients:

- 1 cup snow peas or snap peas
- 2 tablespoons low-sodium soy sauce
- 1 tablespoon rice vinegar
- 1 teaspoon honey
- 1/4 teaspoon red pepper flakes (optional)
- 2 cups cooked brown rice
- 1 lb boneless, skinless chicken breasts, cut into 1-inch pieces
- 2 tablespoons sesame oil
- 2 cloves garlic, minced
- 1 tablespoon grated fresh ginger
- 1 red bell pepper, sliced
- 1 cup broccoli florets
- 1 cup sliced mushrooms

Instructions:

1. In a large skillet or wok, heat the sesame oil over medium-high heat.

2. Add the chicken and stir-fry for 3-4 minutes, or until the chicken is lightly browned.

3. Add the garlic and ginger to the skillet and stir-fry for 1 minute, until fragrant.

4. Add the sliced bell pepper, broccoli, mushrooms, and snow peas or snap peas. Stir-fry for 5-7 minutes, or until the vegetables are tender-crisp.

5. In a small bowl, whisk together the soy sauce, rice vinegar, honey, and red pepper flakes (if using).

6. Pour the soy sauce mixture into the skillet and toss everything together to coat the chicken and vegetables. Serve the chicken and veggie stir-fry over the cooked brown rice.

This chicken and veggie stir-fry is a great option for a PCOS fertility diet for several reasons:

1. Chicken: Chicken is a lean protein source that can help support muscle development and overall health.

2. Vegetables: The bell pepper, broccoli, mushrooms, and snow peas or snap peas provide a variety of vitamins, minerals, and antioxidants that can support fertility and overall health.

3. Brown rice: Brown rice is a whole grain that is a good source of fiber, vitamins, and minerals, which are important for fertility.

4. Healthy fats: The sesame oil provides healthy monounsaturated fats that can help support hormone balance and fertility.

5. Spices and herbs: The garlic, ginger, and optional red pepper flakes add flavor and may also have anti-inflammatory properties that can be beneficial for women with PCOS.

94. Baked Tilapia with Lemon and Garlic

Ingredients:
- 4 tilapia fillets (about 1 lb total)
- 2 tablespoons olive oil
- 2 cloves garlic, minced
- 1 tablespoon fresh lemon juice
- 1 teaspoon grated lemon zest
- 1/4 teaspoon salt
- 1/4 teaspoon black pepper
- 2 tablespoons chopped fresh parsley (optional)

Instructions:
1. Preheat your oven to 400°F (200°C).

2. In a small bowl, combine the olive oil, minced garlic, lemon juice, lemon zest, salt, and black pepper. Mix well.

3. Place the tilapia fillets in a baking dish and pour the lemon-garlic mixture over the top, making sure to evenly coat the fish.

4. Bake the tilapia for 15-20 minutes, or until the fish flakes easily with a fork and is opaque throughout. Sprinkle the baked tilapia with the chopped fresh parsley (if using) before serving.

This baked tilapia with lemon and garlic is a great option for a PCOS fertility diet for several reasons:

1. Tilapia: Tilapia is a lean, mild-flavored fish that is a good source of protein, omega-3 fatty acids, and various vitamins and minerals that are important for fertility.

2. Lemon: Lemon is a good source of vitamin C, which can help support the immune system and overall health.

3. Garlic: Garlic has anti-inflammatory properties that can be beneficial for women with PCOS.

4. Olive oil: The olive oil provides healthy monounsaturated fats that can help support hormone balance and fertility.

5. Parsley (optional): Parsley is a herb that contains antioxidants and may have anti-inflammatory effects that can be helpful for PCOS.

95. Butternut Squash Risotto

Ingredients:
- 1 cup diced butternut squash
- 1 tablespoon olive oil
- 1 onion, diced
- 2 cloves garlic, minced
- 1 cup Arborio rice
- 1/2 cup dry white wine
- 4 cups low-sodium vegetable or chicken broth, heated
- 1/4 cup grated Parmesan cheese
- 2 tablespoons chopped fresh sage
- 1/4 teaspoon salt
- 1/4 teaspoon black pepper

Instructions:

1. Preheat your oven to 400°F (200°C).

2. Toss the diced butternut squash with 1 tablespoon of olive oil and spread it on a baking sheet. Roast for 20-25 minutes, or until the squash is tender and lightly caramelized.

3. In a large saucepan, heat 1 tablespoon of olive oil over medium heat. Add the diced onion and sauté for 3-4 minutes, until translucent.

4. Add the minced garlic and Arborio rice to the saucepan. Stir to coat the rice with the oil and cook for 1-2 minutes.

5. Pour in the white wine and stir constantly until the wine is absorbed, about 2-3 minutes.

6. Add the heated broth to the saucepan, 1/2 cup at a time, stirring constantly until the liquid is absorbed before adding more. Continue this process for 18-20 minutes, or until the rice is tender and creamy.

7. Stir in the roasted butternut squash, Parmesan cheese, chopped sage, salt, and black pepper. Serve the butternut squash risotto warm.

This butternut squash risotto is a great option for a PCOS fertility diet for several reasons:

1. Butternut squash: Butternut squash is a good source of complex carbohydrates, fiber, and various vitamins and minerals, including beta-carotene, which can support fertility.

2. Arborio rice: Arborio rice is a short-grain rice that becomes creamy and tender when cooked, providing a satisfying texture.

3. Parmesan cheese: Parmesan cheese is a good source of protein and calcium, both of which are important for fertility.

96. Moroccan Chickpea Stew

Ingredients:
- 1 tablespoon olive oil
- 1 onion, diced
- 3 cloves garlic, minced
- 1 tablespoon grated fresh ginger
- 1 teaspoon ground cumin
- 1 teaspoon ground coriander
- 1/2 teaspoon ground cinnamon
- 1/4 teaspoon cayenne pepper (or to taste)
- 1 (15 oz) can diced tomatoes
- 1 (15 oz) can chickpeas, drained and rinsed
- 1 cup low-sodium vegetable or chicken broth
- 1 cup chopped cauliflower florets
- 1/2 cup chopped fresh cilantro
- 1/4 cup chopped fresh parsley
- 1 tablespoon lemon juice
- Salt and black pepper to taste

Instructions:

1. In a large saucepan or Dutch oven, heat the olive oil over medium heat.

2. Add the diced onion and sauté for 3-4 minutes, until translucent.

3. Stir in the minced garlic, grated ginger, cumin, coriander, cinnamon, and cayenne pepper. Cook for 1 minute, until fragrant.

4. Add the diced tomatoes, drained and rinsed chickpeas, broth, and chopped cauliflower florets. Bring the mixture to a simmer.

5. Reduce the heat to low and let the stew simmer for 15-20 minutes, or until the cauliflower is tender.

6. Stir in the chopped cilantro, parsley, and lemon juice. Season with salt and black pepper to taste. Serve the Moroccan chickpea stew warm, over cooked quinoa or brown rice if desired.

This Moroccan chickpea stew is a great option for a PCOS fertility diet for several reasons:
1. Chickpeas: Chickpeas are a good source of plant-based protein, fiber, and complex carbohydrates, which can help manage blood sugar levels and support fertility.

2. Cauliflower: Cauliflower is a nutrient-dense vegetable that provides fiber, vitamins, and antioxidants that can support overall health and fertility.

3. Spices: The cumin, coriander, cinnamon, and cayenne pepper add flavor and may have anti-inflammatory properties that can be beneficial for women with PCOS.

4. Herbs: The fresh cilantro and parsley provide additional antioxidants and anti-inflammatory compounds that can support fertility.

97. Seared Tuna with Sesame Seeds

Ingredients:
- 4 (6 oz) tuna steaks
- 2 tbsp sesame seeds
- 1 tbsp coconut or avocado oil
- 2 tbsp reduced-sodium soy sauce or coconut aminos
- 1 tsp rice vinegar
- 1 tsp sesame oil
- 1 tsp freshly grated ginger
- 2 green onions, thinly sliced
- Salt and pepper to taste

Instructions:

1. Pat the tuna steaks dry and season both sides with salt and pepper.

2. Toast the sesame seeds in a dry skillet over medium heat until lightly golden, stirring frequently. Transfer to a shallow dish.

3. Dredge the tuna steaks in the sesame seeds to coat both sides.

4. Heat the coconut/avocado oil in a skillet or grill pan over high heat.

5. Add the sesame seed coated tuna and sear for 1-2 minutes per side for rare, adjusting time for more well-done if desired.

6. In a small bowl, whisk together the soy sauce/coconut aminos, rice vinegar, sesame oil and grated ginger.

7. Transfer the seared tuna to plates and drizzle with the sauce mixture.

8. Garnish with sliced green onions.

This dish is high in protein from the tuna and healthy fats from the sesame seeds and oils. It's gluten-free, dairy-free and low in carbs, making it an ideal main course for a PCOS fertility diet.

98. Turkey and Vegetable Stuffed Peppers

Ingredients:
- 6 bell peppers, tops cut off and seeded
- 1 tbsp olive oil
- 1 lb lean ground turkey
- 1 small onion, diced
- 2 cloves garlic, minced
- 1 cup cooked quinoa or brown rice
- 1 cup diced zucchini
- 1 cup diced mushrooms
- 1 cup diced tomatoes
- 1 tsp dried basil
- 1 tsp dried oregano
- Salt and pepper to taste

Instructions:

1. Preheat oven to 375°F. Lightly oil a baking dish and arrange hollowed out bell pepper halves in the dish.

2. In a skillet, heat the olive oil over medium-high heat. Add the ground turkey and onions. Cook until turkey is browned and onions are translucent.

3. Add the garlic and cook for 1 minute until fragrant.

4. Stir in the cooked quinoa/rice, zucchini, mushrooms, tomatoes, basil, oregano and season with salt and pepper to taste.

5. Stuff each bell pepper cavity with the turkey-vegetable mixture.

6. Cover with foil and bake for 30 minutes. Uncover and bake 15 minutes more until peppers are tender.

7. Let cool slightly before serving. Garnish with fresh parsley or basil if desired.

These stuffed peppers provide a balanced meal of lean protein from turkey, fiber from vegetables and whole grains. They are gluten-free, dairy-free and can be made ahead for an easy, portable PCOS-friendly meal.

99. Spinach and Ricotta Stuffed Shells

Ingredients:
- 20 jumbo pasta shells
- 10 oz frozen chopped spinach, thawed and drained
- 15 oz low-fat ricotta cheese
- 1 egg
- 1/2 cup grated parmesan cheese
- 1 garlic clove, minced
- 1 tsp dried basil
- 1/4 tsp ground nutmeg
- Salt and pepper to taste
- 24 oz jarred marinara or arrabiata sauce
- 1/2 cup shredded mozzarella cheese

Instructions:

1. Cook the jumbo pasta shells according to package instructions until al dente. Drain and rinse with cold water to stop cooking. Set aside.

2. In a bowl, mix together the thawed, drained spinach, ricotta, egg, 1/4 cup of the parmesan, garlic, basil, nutmeg and season with salt and pepper.

3. Spread 1 cup of the marinara sauce in the bottom of a 9x13 baking dish.

4. Stuff each cooked shell with a heaping tablespoon of the spinach-ricotta mixture.

5. Arrange the stuffed shells in the baking dish and top with the remaining marinara sauce.

6. Sprinkle the mozzarella and remaining 1/4 cup parmesan over the top.

7. Cover with foil and bake at 375°F for 25 minutes.

8. Remove foil and bake 10 more minutes until hot and bubbly.

This baked pasta dish is high in protein from the ricotta and parmesan cheeses. The spinach provides fiber, vitamins and minerals. Serve with a side salad for a complete PCOS-friendly meal. You can also make it ahead and refrigerate or freeze for meal prep.

100. Grilled Shrimp with Quinoa Salad

Ingredients:
- 1 lb large shrimp, peeled and deveined
- 2 tbsp olive oil, divided
- 2 cloves garlic, minced
- 1 tsp paprika
- Salt and pepper to taste
- 1 cup quinoa, rinsed
- 2 cups vegetable or chicken broth
- 1 cucumber, diced
- 1 cup cherry tomatoes, halved
- 1/4 cup chopped parsley
- 2 tbsp lemon juice
- 2 tbsp olive oil
- Salt and pepper to taste

Instructions:

1. Toss the shrimp with 1 tbsp olive oil, garlic, paprika, and salt and pepper. Let marinate for 15 minutes.

2. Cook the quinoa according to package instructions, using the broth instead of water.

3. Thread the shrimp onto skewers. Grill over medium-high heat for 2-3 minutes per side until opaque and cooked through.

4. In a large bowl, mix together the cooked quinoa, cucumber, tomatoes, and parsley.

5. In a small bowl, whisk together the remaining 2 tbsp olive oil, lemon juice, and salt and pepper to taste.

6. Pour the lemon dressing over the quinoa salad and toss gently to coat.

7. Serve the grilled shrimp over the quinoa salad.

This light yet filling dish provides lean protein from the shrimp, fiber from the quinoa and vegetables, and healthy fats from olive oil and nuts. It's gluten-free, nutrient-dense and suitable for a PCOS fertility diet. Enjoy it warm or chilled.

101. Greek Yogurt Popsicles with Berries

Ingredients:
- 2 cups plain Greek yogurt
- 1/4 cup honey (or maple syrup for vegan option)
- 1 tsp vanilla extract
- 1 cup mixed berries (strawberries, blueberries, raspberries)

Instructions:

1. In a medium bowl, whisk together the Greek yogurt, honey/maple syrup, and vanilla until well combined.

2. Gently fold in 3/4 of the mixed berries, leaving some for the top of the popsicles.

3. Pour the yogurt mixture into popsicle molds, filling them about 3/4 full.

4. Top each popsicle with some of the remaining berries.

5. Insert popsicle sticks and freeze for at least 4 hours until completely frozen.

6. To remove popsicles, run the molds briefly under warm water to loosen them. Enjoy!

These creamy popsicles make a refreshing, high-protein treat. Greek yogurt provides protein to support fertility. The berries add fiber, vitamins and antioxidants. Honey adds just a touch of sweetness without spiking blood sugar levels.

You can get creative with mix-in ideas like cinnamon, lemon zest, nut butters or different fruits. These popsicles are gluten-free, relatively low in carbs and a perfect snack for a PCOS fertility diet. Enjoy them guilt-free!

102. Banana Oat Cookies

Ingredients:
- 2 ripe bananas, mashed
- 1 cup rolled oats
- 1/2 cup almond flour
- 1/4 cup ground flaxseed
- 1 tsp baking powder
- 1 tsp cinnamon
- 1/4 tsp salt
- 1/4 cup unsweetened almond milk
- 2 tbsp maple syrup (optional)
- 1 tsp vanilla extract
- 1/2 cup walnuts or pecans, chopped (optional)

Instructions:

1. Preheat oven to 350°F. Line a baking sheet with parchment paper.

2. In a large bowl, mash the ripe bananas well with a fork.

3. Add in the rolled oats, almond flour, ground flaxseed, baking powder, cinnamon, and salt. Stir to combine.

4. Pour in the almond milk, maple syrup (if using), and vanilla extract. Mix until a sticky dough forms.

5. Fold in the chopped nuts, if using.

6. Scoop rounds of dough onto the prepared baking sheet, flattening them slightly with a fork.

7. Bake for 15-18 minutes until lightly browned on the edges.

8. Allow cookies to cool on the baking sheet for 5 minutes before transferring to a wire rack.

These flourless banana oat cookies are nutrient-dense and perfect for a PCOS fertility diet. The oats and nuts provide fiber, while the bananas offer natural sweetness. Ground flaxseed is rich in omega-3s. Enjoy these for a filling breakfast or snack. They are gluten-free, dairy-free and have no added sugars.

103. Mango Sorbet

Ingredients:
- 4 cups frozen mango chunks (about 4 large mangoes)
- 1/2 cup unsweetened almond milk
- 2 tbsp honey (or maple syrup for vegan option)
- 1 tbsp fresh lime juice
- 1/4 tsp ground cardamom (optional)

Instructions:

1. Place the frozen mango chunks in a food processor or high-powered blender.

2. Add the almond milk, honey/maple syrup, lime juice, and cardamom (if using).

3. Blend continuously, scraping down sides as needed, until the mixture is smooth and creamy and no chunks remain. This may take 3-5 minutes.

4. Once well blended, scoop the sorbet into an airtight freezer-safe container. Cover surface with wax paper or plastic wrap.

5. Freeze for at least 2 hours before serving to allow it to firm up more.

6. Scoop sorbet into bowls or cups. Allow to sit at room temperature for 5 minutes before eating for optimal texture.

7. Garnish with extra lime zest, chopped mango or mint if desired.

This refreshing mango sorbet is dairy-free, low in carbs and packed with vitamin C and fiber from the fresh mangoes. Honey provides a touch of sweetness without spiking blood sugar levels. It makes a great warm-weather dessert or snack on a PCOS fertility diet. The cardamom adds warmth but can be omitted if desired.

104. Dark Chocolate Bark with Nuts and Seeds

Ingredients:
- 8 oz good quality dark chocolate (70% cacao or higher)
- 1/4 cup raw almonds, coarsely chopped
- 1/4 cup raw walnuts, coarsely chopped
- 2 tbsp pumpkin seeds
- 2 tbsp sunflower seeds
- 1 tbsp chia seeds
- 1 tbsp flaxseeds
- 1/4 tsp sea salt

Instructions:

1. Line a small baking sheet or plate with parchment paper or a silicone mat.

2. Finely chop or break apart the dark chocolate into smaller pieces and place in a microwave-safe bowl.

3. Microwave the chocolate in 30 second intervals, stirring between each, until just melted and smooth.

4. Add in the chopped nuts, seeds, and sea salt. Gently fold to combine them into the melted chocolate.

5. Pour the chocolate-nut mixture onto the prepared baking sheet and spread it out into a thin, even layer using a spatula or knife.

6. Refrigerate for 1-2 hours until the chocolate is completely set.

7. Break or cut the bark into pieces and enjoy! Store leftovers in an airtight container in the fridge.

This dark chocolate bark makes a delicious and healthy treat for women on a PCOS fertility diet. Dark chocolate is rich in antioxidants, while the nuts and seeds provide fiber, protein, and healthy fats like omega-3s. A small amount also has minerals like zinc that support reproductive health.

You can customize it with your favorite nuts and seeds or add dried fruit like goji berries or tart cherries. Enjoy in moderation as part of an overall balanced diet.

105. Almond Milk Ice Cream

Ingredients:
- 2 cups unsweetened almond milk
- 1/2 cup full-fat canned coconut milk
- 1/3 cup honey (or maple syrup for vegan)
- 1 tsp vanilla extract
- 1/4 tsp ground cinnamon
- 1/8 tsp xanthan gum (optional for better texture)
- 1/2 cup raw almonds, toasted and chopped

Instructions:

1. In a blender, combine the almond milk, coconut milk, honey, vanilla, cinnamon and xanthan gum if using. Blend until fully combined and slightly thickened.

2. Pour the mixture into an ice cream maker and churn according to manufacturer's instructions, about 20-25 minutes.

3. During the last 5 minutes of churning, add in the toasted chopped almonds.

4. Once churned, transfer the ice cream to an airtight freezer-safe container. Cover surface with wax paper or parchment to prevent icing.

5. Freeze for at least 2 hours before scooping to allow it to firm up completely.

6. Scoop into bowls or cones. Allow to sit at room temperature for 5 minutes before serving for ideal texture.

This dairy-free, egg-free ice cream is rich and creamy thanks to the coconut milk. Almond milk provides a nutty base. Honey adds just enough sweetness without spiking blood sugar. The almonds give it a delicious crunch.

This version is low in carbs and high in healthy fats, fiber and antioxidants - perfect for a PCOS fertility diet. Feel free to experiment with adding other mix-ins like cacao nibs or your favorite fruits.

106. Pears Poached in Red Wine

Ingredients:
- 4 ripe pears, peeled with stems intact
- 1 bottle (750ml) dry red wine (choose a lighter variety like Pinot Noir)
- ¼ cup honey
- 1 cinnamon stick
- 2 star anise
- 2 cardamom pods, lightly crushed
- 1 vanilla bean, split lengthwise
- Zest of 1 orange

Instructions:

1. Using a melon baller or small spoon, core the pears from the bottom, leaving the stem intact. Set aside.

2. In a large saucepan, combine the red wine, honey, cinnamon stick, star anise, cardamom pods, vanilla bean and orange zest.

3. Add the peeled pears to the wine mixture, stem-side up. The pears should be mostly submerged.

4. Bring the liquid to a gentle simmer over medium heat. Once simmering, reduce heat to low, cover and poach for 15-20 minutes until pears are fork-tender but still holding their shape.

5. Use a slotted spoon to carefully transfer the poached pears to a plate or shallow bowl.

6. Return the poaching liquid to medium-high heat and simmer for 10-15 minutes until reduced and slightly syrupy.

7. Remove whole spices from the reduced syrup. Pour over the poached pears.

8. Allow pears to cool slightly before serving warm, at room temperature, or chilled. Drizzle with extra syrup from the pan.

These fragrant, wine-poached pears make an elegant and flavorful dessert for a PCOS diet. The pears provide fiber, while the red wine adds antioxidants. Honey gives just a touch of sweetness without spiking blood sugar levels. Enjoy them on their own or with a dollop of greek yogurt if desired.

107. Cashew Cheesecake

Crust:
- 1 cup raw almonds
- 1 cup pitted dates
- 1/4 tsp salt

Filling:
- 2 cups raw cashews, soaked in water 4-6 hours, drained
- 1/2 cup coconut cream (from a can of full-fat coconut milk)
- 1/2 cup maple syrup
- 1/3 cup lemon juice
- 1 tsp vanilla extract
- 1/4 tsp salt

Instructions:
For the Crust:
1. In a food processor, pulse the almonds until crumbly. Add dates and salt, pulse until a sticky dough forms.

2. Press the dough into a 7-inch springform pan to form a crust. Refrigerate while making filling.

For the Filling:

3. Blend the soaked cashews, coconut cream, maple syrup, lemon juice, vanilla and salt in a high-speed blender until completely smooth and creamy.

4. Pour the filling over the crust and spread it evenly.

5. Freeze for at least 6 hours until completely set.

6. Before serving, allow to sit at room temperature for 15 minutes. Run a knife around the edges and release the springform ring.. Garnish with fresh berries or lemon zest if desired.

This rich, creamy cashew cheesecake is dairy-free, gluten-free and contains no refined sugars making it perfect for a PCOS fertility diet. The cashews provide protein, healthy fats and minerals like zinc that support reproductive health. The dates in the crust add fiber and natural sweetness.

Allow plenty of time for soaking the cashews and freezing the cheesecake, but the simple preparation is well worth it! Enjoy this decadent dessert in moderation.

108. Cinnamon Baked Pears

Ingredients:
- 4 ripe pears (Bosc or Anjou work well)
- 1 tbsp lemon juice
- 2 tbsp honey
- 1 tsp ground cinnamon
- 1/4 tsp ground ginger
- 1/4 tsp vanilla extract
- 1 cup water or unsweetened almond milk

Instructions:

1. Preheat oven to 375°F (190°C). Grease a baking dish with a little oil or cooking spray.

2. Cut the pears in half lengthwise and use a spoon or melon baller to scoop out the core and seeds, leaving a small well.

3. Arrange the pear halves cut-side up in the prepared baking dish.

4. In a small bowl, whisk together the lemon juice, honey, cinnamon, ginger and vanilla.

5. Brush or spoon the cinnamon-honey mixture evenly over the tops and into the wells of the pear halves.

6. Pour the water or almond milk into the bottom of the baking dish.

7. Cover the dish loosely with foil and bake for 30 minutes.

8. Remove foil and continue baking for 15-20 more minutes until pears are very tender when pierced with a fork.

9. Remove from oven and baste the pears with the cooking liquid once more.

10. Serve the warm baked pears with any remaining sauce spooned over the top. Add a dollop of Greek yogurt if desired.

These baked cinnamon pears make a simple, cozy dessert for a PCOS fertility diet. The pears themselves provide fiber, while the honey gives just a hint of sweetness balanced by warming spices like cinnamon and ginger. This recipe is gluten-free, dairy-free and has no refined sugars. Enjoy after a lighter meal.

109. Raspberry Chia Jam with Greek Yogurt

Ingredients:
- 2 cups fresh or frozen raspberries
- 2 tbsp chia seeds
- 2 tbsp honey (or maple syrup for vegan)
- 1 tbsp lemon juice
- 1 tsp vanilla extract
- Plain Greek yogurt, for serving

Instructions:

1. In a saucepan, combine the raspberries, chia seeds, honey/maple syrup, lemon juice and vanilla extract.

2. Use a potato masher or fork to lightly mash about half of the raspberry mixture, leaving some berries whole.

3. Cook over medium heat, stirring frequently, until the raspberry mixture begins to gently simmer and thicken, about 5-7 minutes.

4. Remove from heat and allow to cool completely, at least 30 minutes. The chia seeds will continue to thicken the jam as it cools.

5. Spoon or transfer the cooled raspberry chia jam into an airtight container and refrigerate until ready to use.

6. To serve, scoop some plain Greek yogurt into a bowl and top with a dollop of the raspberry chia jam.

This simple raspberry chia jam is sweetened naturally with just a touch of honey. The chia seeds provide fiber, protein and healthy omega-3 fats. Paired with Greek yogurt, it makes a protein-packed, antioxidant-rich breakfast or snack perfect for a PCOS fertility diet.

The jam can be made ahead and keeps well refrigerated for up to 1 week. Try swapping in other berries like strawberries or blueberries. Enjoy on yogurt, oatmeal, whole grain toast or on its own!

110. Coconut Macaroons

Ingredients:
- 2 egg whites
- 1/4 cup honey
- 1 tsp vanilla extract
- 1/4 tsp salt
- 2 cups unsweetened shredded coconut
- 2 tbsp coconut flour
- 1/2 tsp cinnamon (optional)

Instructions:

1. Preheat oven to 325°F (165°C). Line a baking sheet with parchment paper.

2. In a medium bowl, whisk together the egg whites and honey until well combined.

3. Stir in the vanilla and salt.

4. Add the shredded coconut, coconut flour and cinnamon (if using). Mix until well incorporated.

5. Using a small cookie scoop or spoon, scoop mounds of the coconut mixture and place them spaced apart on the prepared baking sheet.

6. Bake for 15-18 minutes until lightly golden brown on the tops and edges.

7. Allow macaroons to cool on the baking sheet for 5 minutes before transferring to a wire rack to cool completely.

These chewy, lightly sweetened coconut macaroons get their subtle sweetness from honey instead of refined sugar. The coconut provides healthy fats and fiber. Egg whites give them a chewy texture.

Coconut macaroons are gluten-free, grain-free and dairy-free, making them a great option for a PCOS fertility diet. They are also relatively low in carbs compared to other cookie recipes.

Try dipping the bottoms in melted dark chocolate for an extra special treat, or add some shredded lime or lemon zest to the batter for a citrusy twist! Enjoy in moderation.

As you reach the end of the *"**PCOS Fertility Diet Cookbook for Women: Nutrient-Rich Meals for Balancing Hormones and Enhancing Fertility,**" it is our hope that you feel empowered and inspired to take charge of your health through the power of nutrition. Managing PCOS can be a complex journey, but armed with the right knowledge and tools, you can make meaningful changes that support your well-being and enhance your fertility.*

Throughout this book, we have explored the intricate relationship between diet and PCOS, emphasizing how specific foods and nutrients can play a pivotal role in balancing hormones, improving insulin sensitivity, and promoting reproductive health. The recipes provided have been thoughtfully crafted to not only nourish your body but also delight your palate, making healthy eating an enjoyable and sustainable part of your daily life.

By incorporating these nutrient-rich meals into your routine, you are taking proactive steps toward managing your PCOS symptoms. The emphasis on whole, unprocessed foods ensures that you are fueling your body with the vitamins, minerals, and antioxidants it needs to function optimally. The diverse range of recipes also ensures that you can find meals that suit your taste preferences and lifestyle, making it easier to stick to a balanced diet.

We understand that living with PCOS can sometimes feel overwhelming, but remember that small, consistent changes can lead to significant improvements in your health. This cookbook is designed to be a resource that you can return to time and again, whether you need a new recipe idea, a reminder of the nutritional benefits of certain foods, or simply some encouragement on your journey.

Beyond the recipes, we hope you have found valuable insights and practical tips that will help you make informed choices about your diet and lifestyle. Knowledge is a powerful tool, and understanding how different foods affect your body is a crucial step in managing PCOS and enhancing your fertility.

As you continue on your journey, keep in mind that every individual is unique, and it may take some time to find what works best for you. Be patient with yourself and celebrate the progress you make, no matter how small it may seem. Consistency and dedication to a healthy lifestyle will pay off in the long run.

Thank you for allowing this cookbook to be a part of your journey. We hope it has provided you with the guidance and inspiration you need to make positive changes in your life. Remember, you have the power to take control of your health and well-being. Wishing you all the best in your journey toward balanced hormones, enhanced fertility, and a healthier, happier you.